THE EQUATION OF LIFE

Is there such a thing as a miracle nutrient?

Coenzyme Q_{10} may be the answer.

Oxygen, water, vitamins, proteins, carbohydrates, and fats are all essential to life. You could not live for more than a few minutes without oxygen, more than a few days without water, more than a few weeks without food. It is also true that the body can't survive without Coenzyme Q_{10}. If body levels of CoQ start dropping, so does your general health. A simple equation would read $CoQ_{10} = energy = life$. The following chapters outline exactly what happens when the human body finds itself without sufficient CoQ and how internal supplies of CoQ can be boosted, and your immune system fortified, simply by adding supplements of the coenzyme to your regular diet.

The Miracle Nutrient: Coenzyme Q_{10}

■

Emile G. Bliznakov, M.D.
and
Gerald L. Hunt

BANTAM BOOKS
NEW YORK · TORONTO · LONDON · SYDNEY · AUCKLAND

THE MIRACLE NUTRIENT:
COENZYME Q_{10}
A Bantam Book / January 1987
9 printings through January 1989

Grateful acknowledgment is made to the following for permission to reprint previously published material:
Plenum Publishing Corporation, "New Concepts on the Role of Ubiquinone in the Mitochondrial Respiratory Chain," by Trumpower, B. from J. Bioeng. Bio. Membr. (1981)

Charts courtesy of Elsevier/North-Holland Biomedical Press

ISBN 978-0-553-76313-3

Published simultaneously in the United States and Canada

Bantam Books are published by Bantam Books, a division of Bantam Doubleday Dell Publishing Group, Inc. Its trademark, consisting of the words "Bantam Books" and the portrayal of a rooster, is Registered in U.S. Patent and Trademark Office and in other countries. Marca Registrada. Bantam Books, 666 Fifth Avenue, New York, New York 10103.

PRINTED IN THE UNITED STATES OF AMERICA

146684614

Dedication

This book is dedicated to L.A.M.,
and
MARGARET and JOHN CARLIN

"The great object of science is to ameliorate the condition of man, by adding to the advantages which he naturally possesses."

Elements of Natural Philosophy, 1808

Acknowledgments

The authors would like to acknowledge foremost the pioneering work of Dr. Karl Folkers, the true "father" of CoQ research in the United States, Europe, and Japan. His intrepid and unfailing pursuit of the wonders of coenzyme Q, through his excellence of research and scientific astuteness, has been a model of inspiration for everybody in the field. Without Karl Folkers's endless contributions to the wealth of present knowledge of CoQ, and his constant urging of others to recognize the potential of this nutrient, it is likely that CoQ research would still be in its infancy today.

We would like to thank the National Institute on Aging, the National Institute of Allergy and Infectious Disease, the National Heart, Lung, and Blood Institute, the National Cancer Institute, the American Heart Association, and the American Dental Association for their informational help. Appreciation is also expressed to the Food and Drug Administration for providing information.

We would also like to thank the staff of the American Chemical Society News Service, and especially Nancy Enright for her speed and professionalism in supplying literature on CoQ.

These acknowledgments would not be complete without noting our agents Adele Leone and Richard Monaco for their unswerving support, together with our editor at Bantam, Coleen O'Shea, who grasped the health benefits of CoQ when others failed to do so.

Last, but not least, we are also indebted to Mickey Crean for her research help, support, and indulgence during the preparation and writing of the manuscript.

Important Guidance for Readers

The authors must stress the importance of consulting with your family physician before making any nutritional changes to your regular diet. Although Coenzyme Q_{10} has been found to have no side effects during extensive toxicological studies, we point out that it is important that you do not self-medicate. While we have included numerous beneficial effects of CoQ in this book we do not endorse any medical benefits that may be claimed by the distributors of CoQ products in this country. CoQ_{10} is regarded as a dietary factor, and, as a food supplement, should be looked upon strictly as such. We hope that in the near future the Food and Drug Administration will approve CoQ's sale as a prescription drug, and this will be discussed in more detail in the book. You should consult your physician in order to provide a correct diagnosis of any health problem you might have, and only then should CoQ_{10} supplements be considered alone or in combination with other effective drugs.

Contents

INTRODUCTION

.

A Reporter's Notebook
by Gerald L. Hunt

This book is intended for a general audience as well as medical professionals, and because of this we decided to take a different approach to introduce Coenzyme Q_{10} (CoQ_{10})—a layman's point of view.

The aim is to illustrate some of the usual hesitancy and misunderstandings that meet a "new" nutritional substance, which exhibits enormous beneficial effects for health, when it achieves its first major exposure—and to begin to illustrate the claims you will read about CoQ.

When I was introduced to CoQ, I was skeptical. It seemed unlikely that one common compound could have the potential to manifest so many beneficial applications for human health.

At that time, in 1984, I was co-authoring a book, *The Pain-Free Tryptophan Diet*, which was based on the amino acid L-tryptophan and its potential to help chronic pain victims. The power of tryptophan, a purely natural dietary substance, was impressive—the claims for CoQ, another natural substance, seemed, by comparison, to be extraordinary.

A few months later the subject of CoQ came up again. By this time I'd grown to acknowledge the health potential of nutrients and accept that our own natural pharmacology may well be superior to manufactured drugs in handling problems. After all, many modern drugs have their pharmaceutical roots in herbs and natural nutrients that had been available in apothecary shops and medicine shows for centuries.

The point that impressed me about CoQ was the fact that its critical action occurred at the most basic cellular level; it is a nutrient that was necessary to the function of every single cell in the human body. I began to read about CoQ.

The claims made in *Anti-Aging News* about CoQ seemed

1

genuinely exciting: boosts the immune system; increases the strength of the heart without exercise; relieves angina; protects against heart attacks; lowers high blood pressure; reduces weight naturally; and even extends life itself. Interestingly, most of the so-called benefits of CoQ were based on simply adding supplements of the nutrient to the diet.

Next I raised the issue of CoQ and its potential with several medical professionals only to discover that not one of them had any knowledge of the nutrient. Later I contacted the senior research scientists at a Long Island pharmaceutical company which was the exclusive importer of CoQ from Japan, the only country in the world to produce it in quantity. They were, quite naturally, enthusiastic about the coenzyme, but, more important, they had scientific data on hand, which they sent to me.

The scientific papers contained impressive reports on CoQ studies from universities and institutions throughout the world. I discovered, for example, that the previous literature I had read was supported by major medical studies. And at that time well over 10 million people in Japan, almost 10 percent of the entire population, were taking CoQ daily on a therapeutic basis prescribed by physicians. And in clinical trials, involving thousands of individuals, there were no indications that any toxicity was involved with CoQ. It was, it appeared, totally safe.

I learned that CoQ had been discovered in 1957, and that later Dr. Karl Folkers and research colleagues at the University of Texas in Austin, had been the first scientists to identify its crucial importance in human cell respiration and energy production. But now I wondered why had CoQ been sitting on the laboratory shelf for almost three decades?

Of course it hadn't—especially in Japan where the technology to biologically "grow" amino acids and enzymes, inexpensively and in great volume, had been pioneered and later boomed into a major national asset. In Japan, there were 252 commercial preparations of CoQ being supplied by over 80 pharmaceutical companies. The average dosage was 10 milligrams three times daily, and it was most commonly prescribed for mild congestive heart failure.

One review listed 22 articles, involving 572 heart patients who were involved in studies between 1967 and 1976. It showed mild to dramatic improvements in up to 88 percent of the cases. Accordingly, Japanese medical researchers had been studying CoQ for years in universities and hospitals, with remarkable results across the entire human health spectrum.

Although this biochemical compound had been largely ignored in the United States, I decided to propose an article on CoQ to a weekly news magazine, homing in on the periodontal aspects of CoQ treatment. I focused on this aspect because it was middle-of-the-road, was more likely to be easily substantiated with case histories, anecdotal accounts, and visual proof (it's difficult to interview a cardiac patient and look into their heart at the same time), and was a noninvasive therapy that stood more chance of being accepted by a general audience. Also paramount in my mind were the statistics that showed that one in four people in the United States will eventually lose all their teeth to periodontal disease by age 60, and 90 percent of all Americans will suffer from it during their lifetimes. Periodontal disease is a national disaster in the United States. I was commissioned to proceed with the article.

Investigations lead me to Drs. Wilkinson, dentists and brothers, who had pioneered the periodontal studies of CoQ in the mid-seventies while in the U.S. Air Force. They continued them into private practice and worked in association with Dr. Folkers and the University of Texas. The case histories they had amassed during their studies of the beneficial effects of CoQ on the diseased periodontium were convincing, some even dramatic.

They discovered that unlike healthy oral tissue, cells in the tissue of victims of periodontal diseases were markedly deficient in CoQ. Was the lack of CoQ a result of the disease and therefore an effect; or was it part of the cause?

Commercially available supplemental CoQ in capsule or tablet form was added to the diets of people suffering from periodontal conditions. Some results were dramatic: gums that were once diseased and bleeding began to show clinically significant reversals of the disease process.

One case history involved an elderly woman who had not been able to eat solid foods for months because of intense pain. She was a "no hope" case, according to Dr. Edward Wilkinson. But after 14 days of CoQ supplements the pain diminished and she was eating solids. Three months later her gums were a healthy pink and showed an almost complete reversal of the disease state, desquamative gingivitis. There had been no dental therapy other than the addition of CoQ supplements. Other case histories, backed up by clinical "before and after" laboratory tests of tissue samples, also showed the significant beneficial effects of coenzyme Q.

Dr. Edward G. Wilkinson, a periodontal specialist in private practice in Anchorage, Alaska, admitted that during his dental research days with the U.S. Air Force, he had played devil's advocate at the start of the CoQ studies. Dr. Wilkinson recalled, "I started out as a top notch, number one skeptic on CoQ. But I began to see people improve who I never thought would, or could. It was startling at times to see the reversals. There were changes in diseased gum tissue where I never thought it was possible. My initial doubts were proved to be totally wrong."

The early Wilkinson research was followed and reviewed by Dr. Karl Folkers. The researcher confirmed the periodontal findings to me, stressed the importance of the studies of CoQ and the heart, and stated that he expected CoQ to eventually be a standard addition to the American diet, much like vitamins which are now added to most breakfast cereals.

But surprisingly, the public information specialists at the American Dental Association refused to admit any knowledge of CoQ or its periodontal benefits. And periodontal research experts at the National Institutes of Health sounded nonplussed when presented with the facts. But one of the Bethesda scientists admitted, "It sounds just too good to be true. If there are studies available, I can't understand how we don't know about them. If the facts are accurate, this type of research should take priority under one of our grants."

The periodontal article was written and delivered. It included the Wilkinson studies, Dr. Folkers's comments, and a number of the illuminating case histories. For some unknown reason, possibly because of the lack of enthusiasm from the American Dental Association, the article was shelved.

I continued to pursue investigations of CoQ. Reading through scientific papers on CoQ, one name kept appearing: Emile Bliznakov, M.D., a physician and researcher at the New England Institute in Ridgefield, Connecticut, whose pioneering studies had identified the role of CoQ in the immune system and aging. After meeting with Emile Bliznakov and discussing the health implications of CoQ, I became convinced that I had only scratched the surface of its full potential.

A great amount of scientific information on CoQ is now available in medical libraries as more researchers recognize its potential, especially with respect to the human immune system and the heart.

In 1981 at the Third International Symposium on Coenzyme Q, held in Austin, Texas, Dr. Folkers closed the meeting with a reminder that the traditional view of revolutionary new drugs and therapies is not always one of immediate acceptance. He pointed out that some of the commonly accepted therapeutics in medicine were once looked upon by the scientific community with incredulity. He said:

> New and revolutionary treatments of disease, particularly where there has been no treatment of intrinsic biochemical significance, have generally been believable to a few persons and unbelievable and even ridiculous to others before proof of efficacy. I once heard the story of how incredible the first sulfur drug was to the treatment of infection. To treat pneumonia with a chemical was not considered sane. I witnessed the birth of cortisone to treat disease in a medical environment that was substantially unbelieving. Chemists, in conflict with influential medical opinion, solved the advent of vitamin B_{12}. Revolutionary therapy has always been so and perhaps always shall be, for such is the nature of true discovery. It appears that the bioenergetics of CoQ_{10} is remarkable and its potential in medicine is no exception to the history of controversial advances in medicine.

To this date there have been four international scientific symposiums on CoQ, the last one was held at the Max Planck Institute for Biochemistry in Martinsfried, West Germany, in November 1983. Nobel laureate Dr. Adolf Butenandt opened the meeting with these words: "I do hope that this symposium may encourage German biochemists and clinicians to learn more about the fascinating history of coenzyme Q and to take part in the present and future development in this important field."

Dr. Folkers was chairman of the 3-day symposium, and he concluded with the following comments about the effectiveness of CoQ in treating heart disease: "We have heard that patients in advanced cardiac failure, who had only a few months to live, under close medical care, have revealed almost 'miraculous' improvement after treatment with CoQ_{10}, and such is a step of progress in cardiology.

"Proof of effectiveness of CoQ_{10} in cardiology is now known to medical science. Proof of effectiveness of CoQ_{10} in cardiology for a government agency can now be predicted, planned and achieved. Proof of the safety of CoQ_{10} is known. We have heard more here about patients with side effects from blind placebo than from blind CoQ_{10}."

On April 14, 1986, Karl Folkers was honored with the Priestley Medal, the highest award bestowed by the American Chemical Society in recognition of superior accomplishments in chemistry and medicine. It was presented to Dr. Folkers in recognition of his work with Coenzyme Q_{10}, vitamin B_6, and vitamin B_{12}.

In his Priestley Medal address, Dr. Folkers described his work with CoQ and pointed out that he could report that nearly 500 long-term heart patients had been successfully treated with daily oral doses of CoQ. He added that "long-term coenzyme Q_{10} therapy" was a "major advance" in the treatment of resistant myocardial failure that would not respond to conventional medical therapy. To illustrate this, Dr. Folkers displayed a chart that revealed a 75 percent survival rate over 36 months for patients with congestive heart failure who received conventional therapy plus CoQ, compared to a 25 percent survival rate for patients who received conventional therapy only, including digitalis, diuretics, and vasodilators.

Earlier, on August 1, 1985, the *American Journal of Cardiology* carried a study that indicated that CoQ supplements to the diets of cardiac victims suffering from angina pectoris increased their exercise tolerance and diminished the frequency and pain severity of angina attacks.

Whether CoQ is utilized to bolster the immune system, protect against the damaging effects of aging, lose weight, reduce high blood pressure, strengthen a healthy or a weakened heart, or cure periodontal disease, its effectiveness is now being accepted by scientists and researchers.

As for the periodontal article that sparked my initial interest in CoQ, it was picked up by another weekly magazine. I think it's interesting to note that the same publication that was cautious about the claims of CoQ researchers in 1984, ran a headline in May 1985 that read "New Hope for Heart Patients Who Aren't Helped by Ordinary Medicine"—it was, of course, about CoQ_{10}, the heart and immune system miracle.

This explains my involvement with CoQ as a writer. Since my first meeting with Dr. Bliznakov, scientific studies on CoQ have arrived from his medical research counterparts throughout the world—some of them from Soviet block countries where CoQ research is viewed with paramount importance.

While preparing this book we have repeatedly updated our writings in order to include the latest scientific reports on CoQ, but there are hundreds more ongoing research projects and clinical studies involving CoQ. Those results will be for the future.

As co-author on this work my role, under Dr. Bliznakov's guidance, has been to interpret, write, and relate information from the thousands of items of scientific data that have been made available to us. In the following pages, the narrative of this book is Dr. Bliznakov's. In particular I would like to draw the reader's attention to the use of "we" or "our" in the text when referring to Dr. Bliznakov's research and work at the New England Institute: when the "first person" is used, it refers to research conducted personally by Dr. Bliznakov, or to studies he performed together with various scientific colleagues.

CHAPTER 1

•

CoQ—A Miracle Nutrient?

Is there such a thing as a miracle nutrient?

Coenzyme Q_{10} may be one that comes closer to this description than many of the other nutrients that are considered essential for life.

Oxygen is essential for existence in all life forms. So is water. Vitamins are essential, and so are proteins, carbohydrates, and fats—but not necessarily in that order or in equal amounts. Foods are essential because they supply all the essential nutrients. You could not live for more than a few minutes without oxygen, more than a few days without water, or more than a few weeks without food.

It's also a fact that the body couldn't survive without Coenzyme Q_{10}. If the body levels of CoQ start dropping, so does your general health.

Scientists investigating the role of CoQ in human biochemistry have estimated that once the body levels of CoQ become more than 25 percent deficient many disease states start to flourish. These can range from high blood pressure and heart attacks to deficiencies of the immune system and cancer. If the essential levels of CoQ in your body drop much below a 75 percent deficiency, life can no longer be sustained.

The CoQ and Energy Connection

CoQ is a vital catalyst in the creation of the energy that cells need for life. Without CoQ the chain of cellular energy is broken, and without energy, life ceases. The analogy of the biological energy system as an internal combustion engine helps to illustrate the role of CoQ at the cellular level.

Imagine the V-4, V-6, or V-8 engine in an automobile as an individual human cell. For, in fact, every cell is a minute engine, pumping out energy for use in biological functions—whether it's for playing tennis, solving a difficult mental problem, or just keeping the heart pumping while you sleep.

In each cell there are subcellular components called mitochondria. These can be likened to the cylinders in the automobile engine where gasoline is ignited and explodes, resulting in a force that moves the pistons. In turn this energy is relayed to mechanical drives and gears that eventually turn the wheels of the car. In the human machine it is this energy that fuels the entire body.

In this simplistic view of the mitochondria as cylinders in the minute human cellular engine, ignition is necessary to create energy. This energy production, in the body, results from complicated biochemical processes involving what is called the electron transport system of intracellular respiration—a chain of chemical reactions. One of the most important chemicals in this chain is CoQ.

Without CoQ there's no spark, no ignition, no creation of energy. Take the CoQ out of the mitochondria and you have a cell that has as much potential as a V-8 engine without spark plugs. You have, in essence, a dead engine. If a deficiency of CoQ exists, the result is a cellular engine that, in effect, misfires. If a serious deficiency exists, the mitochondrial engine may eventually fail altogether.

Energy is life, and CoQ is a crucial component of the energy cycle and therefore of life itself.

CoQ Beginnings

In 1957 scientist F.L. Crane and his group in the United States extracted from beef heart mitochondria a new compound, coenzyme Q.

The compound was described by Crane as "capable of undergoing reversible oxidation and reduction"—it can add or remove oxygen from a biologically active molecule. The importance of this statement becomes apparent when it is considered that a lack of oxygen can produce a decline in cellular energy, while an overabundance will result in the formation of potentially lethal peroxides.

CoQ is also known as ubiquinone (*yube-i-kwin-own*). It was named ubiquinone by British researcher R. A. Morton, because it is ubiquitous (exists everywhere) in life.

In chemical terms CoQ is a quinone, a member of a group

of brightly colored cyclic organic compounds. Many quinones occur in nature, one of the most important being vitamin K_1, which is used as an antihemorrhagic agent and is found in certain green plants. Among the quinones, one of the most important for industrial use is anthraquinone, which is used as a dyestuff intermediate. Several quinones are biologically important as coenzymes and similar to certain vitamins. An example of an essential substance with a quinonelike chemical structure is vitamin E. The potent anticancer agent Adriamycin also has a structure similar to the quinones.

We know that CoQ is an integral part of the mitochondria, the subcellular components that are responsible for generating about 95 percent of the total energy needed by the human body. CoQ exists in the membranes of mitochondria, from where it performs its critical function, the manufacture of adenosine triphosphate (ATP), the basic energy molecule of the cell.

But CoQ is far more abundant in the cells of some organs than in others. There are high concentrations of CoQ in the organs that need the largest supplies of energy, like the heart and the liver. It is because CoQ plays such a vital role in the production of energy that extra supplies of it are needed in the heart, which is constantly beating; in the liver, which is the powerhouse of human biochemistry; and in the cells of the immune system, which fight off dangerous disease-causing bacterial and viral invaders.

Studies have shown that if the essential levels of CoQ are allowed to decline, and the body's vital organs and systems cannot meet their energy requirements, the inevitable results are major ill health and disease states. Furthermore, with advancing age the body begins to lose its own innate ability to supply CoQ. This can result in deficiencies of CoQ needed to fight off the diseases normally associated with aging.

The Immune System and Aging

One of the most obvious signs of aging is the decrease in the powers of the immune system. Like people who are malnourished or who have diminished immunity through illness or disease, older people are less able to ward off even minor ailments like the common cold. What may be just a cold or influenza for a person with a healthy immune system can result in pneumonia and even death for the elderly. Their immunological functions deteriorate with age to such a point that they are no longer able to fight off illness and infections.

Although today's antibiotics and antiviral drugs can aid the diminished power of the immune system, they cannot cure its deficiencies. The drugs act as reinforcements in the immunological fight, but these biological aids will not help the body's immune system build up additional potential immunity against future attack. Moreover, only so much additional strength can be injected into the immune system, and if the reserves are already too low, little can be done but to stand by and watch the invader take over.

This is the tragedy that overcomes the victims of the controversial disease AIDS (acquired immunodeficiency syndrome). AIDS victims have no immune defenses to fight off invading infections and viruses. In theory even something as minor as a common sore throat could kill an AIDS victim.

Drugs—antibiotics, for example—can help out the immune system when it's under severe stress from infections. Unfortunately the system cannot always rebound after an illness or disease state to create new resistance. But scientists have now discovered that CoQ is an integral part of the immune cycle, when immunity is low, so, it has been discovered, are the reserves of CoQ. When CoQ is boosted, so is the immune potential.

Many of the ill effects of aging can be linked directly to the failing of the immune system. And it is not just coincidence that the decline of the immune potential directly parallels the body's inability to supply CoQ internally.

If we were able to keep the immune system at near peak performance during the advancing years when it normally begins to decline rapidly, could we extend not only the quantity of life but also the quality?

The answer from the laboratory appears to be yes. Experiments with human subjects take many years. The process can be accelerated, however, by using animal models that have a much shorter life span.

In our own experiments with female mice at the New England Institute, the life spans of these animals were increased by some 50 percent and more by simply giving them supplemental CoQ. And, equally fascinating was the fact that the quality of youthful life was noticeably maintained well into the animals' extended life spans.

With these animal models the boosting of CoQ was achieved

by injecting it into their bodies. One of the most noticeable physical features to be observed was that even though the mice had surpassed their normal life schedules, they still had healthy, glossy coats and skin, and showed little or none of the expected signs of aging, like patchy loss of fur, organ degeneration, and lack of mobility. In fact, the last surviving mouse in our experiment lived to 150 weeks—or about 140 years by human standards.

Work on the benefits of CoQ and the immune system has been going on throughout the scientific world. In another area, one of the most intriguing biological discoveries during the past decade was the existence of chemicals known as free radicals. These highly active molecules attack and disrupt the vital chain of oxygen supplies at the cellular level. It is now believed that the free radicals play a significant role in tissue injury, disease states, and, especially, aging.

It has been found that CoQ acts as an antioxidant—it protects the cells against free radicals and maintains their vital oxygen lifeline. And now it has been discovered that there is a vital link between CoQ and vitamin E. Dr. Lars Ernster, of the University of Stockholm, comments on Swedish CoQ research. He confirms, "Ubiquinone exerts effects against free radicals as an antioxidant, similar to vitamin E. In fact there is evidence for a protective effect of ubiquinone against lipid peroxidation that results in serious membrane damage and is also responsible for 'age granules' in aging cells."

Yet another important role of CoQ in the immune and aging processes is now being established. Macrophages are uniquely special cells that play a key role in fighting off immune system invaders. Research at the New England Institute established for the first time that CoQ can act as a stimulating agent for the activation of macrophages.

Many other special cells are essential to the development of cellular and humoral immunocompetence (that is, a strong immune system). CoQ is an immunostimulating agent able to activate a wide range of beneficial functions. Immunostimulating agents (called immunomodulators) also possess power to enhance antibacterial action and even antitumor effects—front line defenses that protect the biological system from attack. But what suggests that CoQ is even more important is that during some pathological states, for example when infections begin to run rampant, or in the aging process itself, scientists have observed CoQ deficiencies. This indicates that CoQ is a crucial component for the optimal functioning of the immune system.

Worldwide clinical tests of CoQ show that the nutrient has far-reaching beneficial implications when used to naturally boost an immune system that is not operating at peak efficiency due to disease or infection, or one that has fallen prey to the ravages of tumors or aging.

The Heart

The heart is the pump of life. A decline in cardiac ability is most often noticed during the later stages of life. The process of degenerative heart disease very rarely strikes before middle age, and when it does it correlates with the diminution of the body's ability to produce its own CoQ.

During early research into CoQ, biochemists proposed a rather radical theory: they believed that CoQ might play a role in the health of cardiac muscle. Researchers began probing into the chemical contents of diseased heart tissue after death to search for clues. The theoretical assumption didn't seem to be quite so radical once a significant lack of CoQ was found in the "tired" cells.

Samples of myocardial tissue biopsies were compared for CoQ content with biopsies from healthy hearts. The differences were impressive. This type of biomedical detective work was followed up with the noninvasive techniques, measuring the levels of CoQ in the blood of cardiac disease victims, and again a significant decline of CoQ was noticed.

When CoQ was administered to heart patients orally as a dietary supplement, failing cardiac systems took on renewed vigor. The main parameters of measurement for heart efficiency, cardiac output and stroke volume, were significantly increased. This showed that the organ had taken a dramatic turn toward better health and away from the degenerative disease process. These benefits were being exhibited in a matter of weeks without the influence or aid of traditional cardiac medications.

When similar doses of CoQ were administered in clinically controlled tests to sufferers of angina pectoris, the same beneficial effects were observed. Angina is an ideal condition to study CoQ because signs of improvement can be observed and measured without having to invade the body to find them.

For some angina victims even the slightest bit of exercise can be intolerable, resulting in the onset of stabbing chest pains. This is a clear indication of the heart's distress and the onset of an angina attack. With CoQ, patients were able to significantly increase their endurance in treadmill tests without discomfort—in some cases being able to double the time they were formerly able to endure on the treadmills.

These results then lead researchers to theorize that the condition of the otherwise healthy but aging myocardium could be improved and protected against the inevitable process of aging.

A good way to strengthen the heart is through aerobic exercise which, over the long term, will improve its performance. But not everybody is willing, or even able, to endure strenuous workouts. Could CoQ be used prophylactically to strengthen the heart of sedentary people?

In experiments in the United States involving volunteers who did not have the benefits of exercise or fitness programs, 60 mg of supplemental CoQ was administered each day to their diets for 8 weeks. In this short time their hearts were able to display an increase in oxygen utilization and their maximal exercise loads improved dramatically. This improvement was achieved without additional exercise of any type.

Another exciting discovery was made involving CoQ and the use of lifesaving cardiac drugs. Researchers found that in serious cases of cardiac distress, when potent drugs had to be used to stabilize the condition, the addition of CoQ supplements allowed physicians to dramatically reduce the drug dosages while still achieving the same therapeutic results.

The distinct advantage of this CoQ-and-drug regimen was that the dosages of the cardiac drugs, many of which have toxic side effects that can have adverse reactions on other organs in the body, could be reduced. When CoQ and cardiac drugs were used in tandem, the drug dosages could be reduced and therefore the unwanted side effects were lower or did not exist at all.

High Blood Pressure

High Blood Pressure is known as the "silent killer" because it goes undetected in the majority of the population.

Hypertension, the name most medical professionals prefer to use, has few, if any, symptoms among the one hundred million people who may be suffering from this disease in the United States. For someone with seriously elevated blood pressure, an eventual diagnosis may even come too late, after most of the damage has been done.

High blood pressure is the disruption of the delicate balance in the force that pumps blood through the veins and arteries. It is known as vascular pressure and when it builds up to unsafe levels it places an undue load on the heart and the entire vascular system leading to vessel failure, stroke, and heart attack.

There are numerous drugs to counteract elevated blood pressure. The first line of medical defense in simple cases of hypertension is usually a diuretic, an agent that rids the body of excess fluid. But even a mild diuretic may have side effects, and when physicians turn to the more potent antihypertensives, the seriousness of side effects increases dramatically.

Diet can also play a major role in controlling high blood pressure, but unless the condition has been diagnosed as life-threatening, many people are not amenable to changes in their nutritional life-style—such as giving up smoking and drinking—for a state of health that exhibits no symptoms. Medical health experts have only started getting tough on hypertension during the last two decades since it was realized that the hypertension problem may turn out to be the nation's number one precursor of cardiac disease states.

Because of the link between hypertension and cardiac mortality, CoQ researchers began to look into the possibility that there was also a link between blood pressure and the coenzyme.

In studies in both the United States and Japan, physicians have lowered the blood pressure of cardiac high risk patients by simply adding CoQ supplements to their diets: a completely natural remedy without additional medication. A typical case study shows: prior to CoQ therapy, average systolic reading 141, diastolic 97. After 2 months of CoQ therapy, average reading, systolic 126, diastolic 90.

CoQ researcher Dr. Philip C. Richardson, of the University of Texas in Austin, believes that CoQ has the potential to be the most effective alternate clinical control of elevated blood pressure, with none of the unwanted side effects of drugs.

Losing Weight Naturally

With all the fad diets, potions and pills, and weight control books on the market today it's no wonder that most people are confused as to which method might work for them. What is true is that weight loss is accomplished when the caloric intake is less than what the body is used to and less than what the body needs. The safe and sensible way to lose weight and maintain weight loss is to gradually lower your intake of calories and increase exercise. It's a matter of literally burning off excess stored energy, which is all that fat deposits are. By stepping up your metabolic needs with exercise, you increase the demand for energy and the body deploys its most immediately accessible energy reserves, which are stored in the fat cells. As the reserves dwindle, so do the contents of the fat cells, and weight loss, through reduced fat supplies, becomes evident.

There is also another way, and that is to increase your metabolic fuel efficiency within the cells. Some scientists believe that this is exactly how weight loss in the obese can be induced by CoQ. A combined study between the University of Texas and the University of Antwerp, in Belgium, has shown that the obese can lose weight with the addition of CoQ to the diet.

The same research revealed that the very obese could display as much as a 50 percent deficiency of CoQ in tissue cells. By comparison, people who eat well, yet remain slim and trim, were found to have significantly higher levels of CoQ in their blood.

To test the theory that supplemental CoQ might aid the obese, a study was conducted and the results showed that the addition of CoQ to the diets of obese people with CoQ deficiencies resulted in weight loss.

Periodontal Disease

As mentioned in the introduction, CoQ's role in periodontal health mirrors its action in the protection and strengthening of the heart, and of the vascular and immune systems. Working from the cellular level it helps promote strong, active, and healthy cells, whether they are in the myocardium or the gums. The lack of CoQ in the periodontal tissues leads to the inevitable decline that is found in other tissues of the body when they are deprived of adequate amount of this essential coenzyme.

Chapter 11 details case histories of patients with even the most severe periodontal disease states who have found relief and renewed oral health with supplements of CoQ.

Too Good to Be True?

These are some of the obvious benefits of CoQ, but there are many more, including its role in fighting cancer; aiding in surgery by protecting the brain and other vital organs; and potentially increasing the chances of survivability of organ transplants.

How can one nutrient do all these things?

When Alexander Fleming first discovered penicillin, other physicians, including his close colleagues in Edinburgh, laughed him out of the lecture hall when he said it could act as a powerful medicine against not just one type of infection, but many. He might have found a more receptive audience if he'd limited his discovery to a cure for sore throats. Today we use penicillin as a potent line of attack against a multitude of bacterial ailments. It was the first antibiotic.

The power of penicillin and other antibiotics that initially went unrecognized was their ability to work at an elemental level throughout the entire body, aiding the immune system in destroying invading microorganisms. CoQ has the power to implement beneficial changes in the immune system, but its action boosts the effectiveness of the immune response, without having a direct effect on the microorganisms. Clearly when antibiotics and CoQ work in tandem a significantly increased beneficial effect can be anticipated, with antibiotics working from the outside through the circulation, and CoQ from within individual cells.

The body's cells are constantly dying and being replaced. CoQ is also essential to all this construction and reconstruction.

In the following chapters the different actions of CoQ in various conditions of human health are explained together with the results of hundreds of clinical and experimental studies that have proven the benefits of CoQ.

CHAPTER 2

•

The CoQ Connection

The story of CoQ is a fascinating tale of biological wonders and even industrial intrigue. In early experiments to show the role of CoQ in the bioenergetics of human life, Dr. Karl Folkers made a dramatic finding. According to his calculations, once our levels of CoQ drop down to 25 percent of our expected norm (a 75 percent deficiency), death can be expected. And once levels of CoQ start falling below 75 percent (a 25 percent deficiency) of our expected norm, numerous kinds of diseases may begin to take hold in the body as a result of the deficiency.

Dr. Folkers stated, "CoQ_{10} is necessary for human life. Morbidity is associated with a deficiency of CoQ_{10} of about 75%, and death may occur somewhere between a deficiency of 75 and 100%. Low tissue deficiencies of CoQ_{10} may be subclinical, but somewhere between 25 and 75% deficiencies, overt disease states may appear."

Most CoQ clinicians now subscribe to this finding, and many believe that Dr. Folkers's original calculations may have been too optimistic, and that serious states of ill health will result with much less of a deficiency than Dr. Folkers first predicted.

The following chapters outline exactly what happens when the human body finds itself without sufficient CoQ. How, for example, the immune system or the heart can be deficient in CoQ and not have the energy to overcome ill health and disease states, and how internal supplies of CoQ can be boosted by simply adding supplements of the coenzyme to the regular diet.

At this point it is most important to bear in mind that it's absolutely essential for sufficient CoQ supplies to be coming into the body to meet the constant demand for energy going out. This energy, created at a molecular subcellular level, is what life is all about. Take away the supply of energy and life force is extinct. A simple equation would read CoQ = energy = life.

How Do We Get CoQ?

Humans obtain CoQ through foods. Everything that was once living, and relied on respiration to produce energy, contains CoQ. Anything that ever breathed has to contain CoQ, because CoQ supplies the energy for respiration.

Plants get CoQ from the soil, the richest chemical depository on earth. The plant's internal pharmaceutical factory pulls the different chemical components together to form a single CoQ specific for that plant.

Microbes also need CoQ to survive. They could get it from the soil they live in, or from the plant or other living matter on which they survive. The fact is that microbes also hold the golden key to how all the commercially available CoQ is produced today for human consumption.

Going up the biological chain, called the food chain, it's easy to see how everything from the smallest microbe to the largest mammal gets its CoQ. The human, at the top of the food chain, eats plants and animals that have already obtained their CoQ from what they fed on further down the chain. One of the richest sources of CoQ as a readily available food is beef heart. CoQ is also contained in the muscles and organs of many animals that we eat, but hearts normally have the richest concentration. Just as the human heart has the highest concentrations of CoQ, so does the heart of the cow.

Every time we eat a steak, a chicken leg, a bowl of cereal, or a green pepper, we are helping to replenish the body's internal stock of CoQ. All these food sources don't, however, contain the same amounts of CoQ.

Anything that ever lived will contain varying amounts of CoQ. If soil does indeed contain all the elements necessary to construct CoQ, wouldn't it make sense to assume that soil would be a rich supplier of CoQ? Yes, but unfortunately the body does not have the ability to fuse together all the chemicals contained in soil to form CoQ. This has to be done for us at lower levels on the food chain. In essence, the CoQ we

receive through our diets is second hand, or a more acceptable way of looking at it might be that CoQ supplies are
"ready made" or "preproduced" for us.

The CoQ Family

There are ten common CoQs, and possibly more still to be
identified and catalogued. They are spread among the life
forms around us, in the plants and animals. The only CoQ of
direct importance to humans is CoQ_{10}.

CoQ is a ubiquinone. Imagine this ubiquinone as a circle of
chemical elements that all combine to form a single CoQ
molecule. This chemical ring is CoQ in its most basic form.

The next step is to add the ingredient that makes one
variety of CoQ different from another. The CoQ molecule has
a side chain that contains carbon atoms—and the more of
these carbon atoms that are attached to the basic CoQ molecule, the larger the number we assign to that variation of
CoQ. Illustrations I and II show CoQ_{10} with its unique side
chain of atoms.

The carbon atoms on the side chain always join together in
groups of five, and a single numeral is assigned to each
cluster. For example, in CoQ_1 there are five atoms in the side
chain. Likewise, in CoQ_2 there are ten atoms; CoQ_6, 30
carbon atoms; and in CoQ_{10}, 50.

Only CoQ_{10} is found in human tissues, CoQ_6 and CoQ_7
have been identified in yeasts, and CoQ_8 in bacteria, such as
Escherichia coli (E. coli). It would seem that the higher up
the evolutionary scale, the higher the CoQ type. But this is
not necessarily so. Mice, for example, have only CoQ_9, while
certain plants, like tobacco, and bacteria, like Micrococcus
glutamicus, contain CoQ_{10}. The latter two examples become
highly significant later in this chapter.

To compound the mystery even further, all vertebrates
have CoQ_{10} and only CoQ_{10}, except for rats, mice, and a
member of the fish family, the walleyed pike, which have
been identified as containing CoQ_9, or CoQ_{10} plus CoQ_9.

This inconsistency is a biological puzzle. There doesn't
seem to be any rationale for why this should be so, and
there's no adequate scientific explanation for it. It just has to
be accepted for now as a fact and a quirk of nature that may
one day be explained fully by scientific investigation.

Illustration I

Coenzyme Q$_{10}$

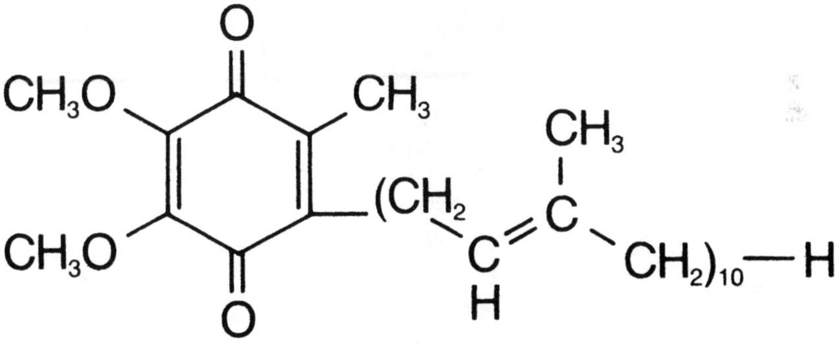

CH_3O — (ring with two $=O$ groups, CH_3, and CH_3O substituents) —$(CH_2\!-\!\underset{H}{C}\!=\!\underset{\underset{CH_3}{|}}{C}\!-\!CH_2)_{10}\!-\!H$

This is Coenzyme Q$_{10}$. Its formation with atoms of oxygen, hydrogen and carbon, together with its unique side chain of 50 atoms—in ten groups of five—distinguishes it from others in the coenzyme Q family. The figure $_{10}$ at the end of the formula indicates that the single unit of the side chain is repeated 10 times.

Illustration II
A Different View of CoQ$_{10}$

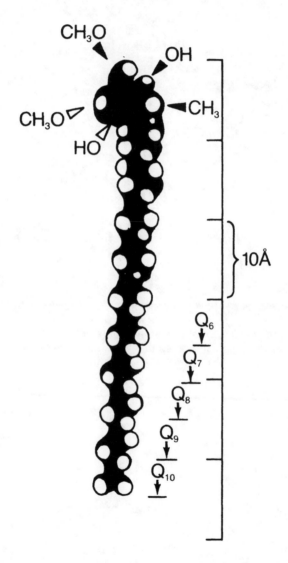

This is a representation of how CoQ$_{10}$ might be viewed in nature at the molecular level. Notice the long side chain leading off from the main molecule (with the cutoff points indicated for other CoQ's). The long length of the side chain is what makes CoQ$_{10}$ so unique among the CoQ family.

The following condensed table lists the naturally occurring ubiquinones.

Source	Ubiquinones
Microorganisms (some)	Q-1 to Q-6
Yeasts	Q-6, Q-7
Bacteria	Q-8, Q-9, Q-10
Plants	Q-9, Q-10
Fungi	Q-7, Q-8, Q-9, Q-10
Invertebrates	Q-9, Q-10
Vertebrates*	Q-10

*Except the rat, mouse, and walleyed pike

In the pioneering days of coenzyme Q, Dr. Karl Folkers isolated the nutrient from human hearts and was one of the first researchers to confirm that the coenzyme in the human was indeed CoQ_{10}. Folkers confirmed, "Since some living species have other forms of functional CoQ, that is Q_6, Q_7, Q_8, and Q_9, it was important to prove for medicine which CoQ is in the human heart. Therefore, CoQ_{10} is the "human Q" and is the one which should be used and is used for clinical research and to treat human disease."

For the sake of brevity throughout this book, when coenzyme Q is referred to without any defining number (i.e., CoQ), it is specifically CoQ_{10}.

How the Other Qs Work for Humans

Human tissue contains only CoQ_{10}. Any lower CoQs just don't have the potential necessary for creating optimal energy within the human system of bioenergetics. But the human body can utilize the other CoQs through the work of chemical conversions that take place in the liver. In the liver the side chain atoms are stripped away from the basic molecule of coenzyme Q and then reassembled and reattached in amounts that add up to CoQ_{10}. It is the failure of this internal alchemy that also dictates why in some people—especially the elderly—deficiencies of CoQ can occur.

Here's a hypothetical meal and a description of how the liver performs this unique processing: The meal is comprised of a mug of beer (because of their brewing processes, tea and coffee will not provide biochemically useful CoQs, but beer will through the yeasts and bacteria in the fermentation process), clams on the half shell, and a side order of any vegetable and mushrooms. Let's say that the yeast in the beer contains six CoQ_6s; the shellfish (invertebrates), eight CoQ_9s; the vegetables (plants), twelve CoQ_9s; and the mushrooms (fungus), nine CoQ_7s.

After the meal has been digested and the different forms of coenzyme Q arrive in the liver, they are broken down so that the whole meal produces 279 single blocks of atoms, which are then recombined to produce only CoQ_{10}s, resulting in 27 new CoQ_{10}s that have been synthesized for our human needs.

If the meal had also contained a piece of steak, for example, we might have had an additional 12 CoQ_{10}s, which would have brought the grand total for the whole meal to 39 CoQ_{10}s.

This, of course, is a gross simplification, the figures given to individual CoQs (which would have to be in atomic and molecular weights) have been used simply as an illustration. No scientist has yet been able to quantify the exact number of CoQ atoms and molecules in any given weight of bacterial, fungous, plant, or animal matter. The process of identifying a given life form and determining which CoQ it contains is still in its infancy. It is, however, enough to confirm at this stage that a specific plant or animal tissue contains an identifiable amount of a specific coenzyme Q.

So, while not all the foods we eat contain the necessary CoQ_{10}, the body can manipulate the others to make CoQ_{10} in the liver. A good balanced diet should ensure that the body won't suffer from a lack of CoQ.

But soon after scientists began finding CoQ deficiencies in people with ill health and in disease states, they began to wonder what could be causing these deficiencies, which were even more noticeable in the elderly. It was discovered that the liver's system of CoQ splicing isn't foolproof and, in fact, this ability was suspected to decline with age. It is unknown at this time why, or how, this takes place.

As we get older, we still utilize the complete CoQ_{10}s we get in our foods, but we are no longer able to produce them from other forms of the CoQs, or cells in the aging organism demand more than we can produce. This can lead to a deficiency of CoQ throughout the entire body.

It becomes very obvious that when the human body might be needing the benefits of CoQ the most, for example when fighting off heart disease or cancer in middle age, or even the process of aging itself, its ability to supply enough CoQ may be severely reduced with age. This is the one single reason why CoQ_{10} supplements may be vital for some people to retain maximum health and fight off the processes of disease and aging.

It has been confirmed in clinical studies involving thousands of people who are in ill health—for example suffering from heart disease or diseases associated with weakened immune response—that if supplements of CoQ are administered, their internal levels of CoQ rise and the disease states diminish as the body acquires renewed energy to fight them off.

Measuring the Body's Levels of CoQ

Samples of blood can be analyzed to give an indication of whether the body has adequate levels of CoQ. As yet, this is a laboratory technique and is not the simple sort of blood workup that can be conducted in the physician's office. The only drawback with a blood analysis is that the blood supplies only a general indication of CoQ levels; it is not specific for each organ. It can reveal a good overview of what is going on in the body, but it doesn't provide a clear-cut picture of the status of the different organs.

Heart tissue, for example, which contains more CoQ than any other organ in the body, may be moderately deficient in CoQ (enough, anyway, to cause a decline in its energy potential and possibly leave it open to disease states), but the blood reading from the entire body may show no significant overall deficency of CoQ. But if a significant decrease of CoQ were discovered in the blood, it would be highly likely that an organ like the heart, with its high call for CoQ, would definitely be in a state of serious CoQ deficiency.

Is CoQ a Vitamin?

The classic description of a vitamin is that it is a substance that is essential to life and that can be acquired only in integral form, through nutrition. A substance is not regarded as a vitamin if it can be synthesized naturally within the body from the chemicals obtained from food sources.

CoQ is therefore an anomaly. It is essential to life, but the CoQ_{10} required by the human body can be produced from other CoQs in the diet—however, the body does not have the ability to synthesize it from the individual chemical building blocks that are bonded together to form CoQ. From this perspective it might not be considered a true vitamin even though the original sources of CoQ are only available through nutrition.

We know that our internal ability to supply CoQ_{10} declines with age, and when this happens the only source of pure CoQ_{10} is directly from foods in the diet that contain it in the CoQ_{10} form. It can be argued that CoQ now meets all the requirements of a true vitamin.

Dr. Karl Folkers states that the scientific qualifying parameters for vitamins need to be urgently reviewed. Under an updated definition by the scientific community, CoQ would undoubtedly be classed as a vitamin.

"CoQ_{10} belongs to the science of nutrition, and is like a vitamin. On occasion, this molecule is called vitamin Q_{10}, but in doing so, one is updating the 70-year-old definition of a vitamin, which required that a vitamin must not be synthesized by mammalian tissue, but be of dietary source," explains Dr. Folkers. He continues, "This old definition of a vitamin should not include ascorbic acid (vitamin C) and nicotinic acid (vitamin B_3), which have long been known as vitamins, because mammalian tissue has the capacity to biosynthesize ascorbic acid and nicotinic acid as well as CoQ_{10}.

"Nomenclature is arbitrary, depending upon the state of the science at the time the nomenclature is created. If ascorbic acid and nicotinic acid may be called vitamins, then Coenzyme Q_{10} may also be called a vitamin. In terms of biochemistry, the designation Coenzyme Q_{10} is better than vitamin Q_{10}, because the substance actually functions as a coenzyme. Many vitamins must be converted to the corresponding coenzymes for functionality."

Dr. Folkers makes the important point that many vitamins are functionally useless as nutrients until they are converted in the body to coenzymes. It could therefore be suggested that CoQ has a status in nutrition that is superior to that of vitamins.

Timing the Benefits of CoQ

An often asked question is: How long will it take before I notice the benefits of CoQ?

First, it has to be understood that additional supplements

of CoQ to the diet will only have a beneficial effect if a deficiency is already present. But, as is explained in Chapter 3 on CoQ and the immune system, it is highly likely that most humans experience deficiencies of CoQ at some points in life—for example, when under stress or during illness and states of immune deficiency—and especially as they grow older.

In a severe state of CoQ deficiency, a person may expect to experience benefits within a few days. The biochemical reason for this may be likened to a sponge absorbing water—the drier the sponge, the more water it will absorb immediately. In the case of a person with a moderate to mild deficiency of CoQ the uptake will be a slower, more gradual process as CoQ levels rise toward the norm.

Explains Dr. Karl Folkers,

On the basis that CoQ_{10} is like a vitamin, it may be expected that the response of a patient with disease to treatment with CoQ_{10} will occur only when the patient has a deficiency of CoQ, which is significant to the disease state. CoQ_{10} is not a drug—it is not a classical medicinal, although it is used like a drug. Therefore, CoQ_{10} does not have a pharmacodynamic activity which appears within minutes, hours, or a day or two, and which is renewed by subsequent dosage.

The therapeutic action of CoQ_{10} is based upon molecular biology, which according to our understanding of today, involves increases in tissue levels of CoQ_{10}-enzymes and saturation by CoQ_{10} of empty receptor sites. The therapeutic effect which is observed with oral CoQ_{10} over one to three months or longer is compatible with knowledge that the translational increases in the levels of such enzymes is a time-requiring process. This means that clinical protocols to evaluate CoQ_{10} must take into account that the mechanism of activity of CoQ_{10} is in bioenergetics.

But there are instances when CoQ's beneficial effects are observed much faster. This can occur when CoQ is utilized together with another drug, either as a protective "buffering" agent to reduce possible side effects, or as a booster to a drug's potential by improving performance at the site it has been aimed at—for example, the immune system.

Is CoQ Safe?

In toxicological tests, involving thousands of human subjects, no risk of toxicity has ever been observed involving CoQ. Unlike a drug being administered into the body, CoQ is completely natural and not a substance that is alien to the human biological machine. No matter how high the dosage of CoQ, no significant toxicity has ever been recorded. And this includes long-term studies over many years.

The only noticeable side effect associated with supplemental oral CoQ—and it must be stressed that this is extremely rare—has been transient mild nausea.

According to the stringent requirements of the Food and Drug Administration (FDA), extensive toxicological tests have to be performed on various types of animals, including mice, rats, rabbits, dogs, and monkeys, before scientists are ever permitted to use the substance on humans. This experimental stage is followed by the next step known as Phase I clinical trials, which involves terminally ill patients (usually with cancer). Only after the FDA is completely satisfied that the new drug has displayed no significant toxic effects will the clinicians be permitted to go to Phase II clinical trials, which then look, for the first time, for the beneficial effects of the new drug.

In material supplied to the FDA from scientific groups, including our own research findings, no toxic effects were observed that would preclude the use of CoQ in humans.

Our studies involving terminal cancer patients, conducted at the Yale Medical School, New Haven, Connecticut, were started in March of 1972 and concluded in 1974. They were then submitted to the FDA and accepted. Phase II clinical trials are now in progress in numerous medical establishments and hospitals throughout the United States, and many are reported on in this book.

These are the strict requirements that apply only for trials in the United States. Other countries have their own various rules, including Japan and West Germany, whose requirements are as thorough as the FDA.

Industrial Intrigue

It may surprise people suffering from potentially fatal heart disease today to learn that a nutrient exhibiting promise of relief and recovery is not well known in the United States, yet millions take it every day in Japan where it's considered a lifesaving medication for cardiac problems. High manufacturing costs are part of the reason why U.S. pharmaceutical companies are not actively involved in the production of CoQ.

During early CoQ research the only reliable source of CoQ was from beef heart. But the availability and costs of production were staggering. The cost of one gram of CoQ from beef heart was about $1,000, and that was in an unpurified state. The entire human body contains a total of 2 grams of pure CoQ_{10}.

Following Dr. Karl Folkers's earliest experiments to prove the efficacy of CoQ, research scientists at Hoffmann-La Roche Company developed and patented a complicated method of chemically synthesizing and producing CoQ in bulk. The cost, however, was even more expensive.

Meanwhile, in the early 1970s, Japanese scientists leaped ahead with a new technology that produced vast amounts of natural CoQ at much less cost. The key to this production breakthrough was tobacco.

Although the chemical process was highly complicated, the researchers had managed to isolate a substance in the tobacco plant that provided the key CoQ_{10} side chain of 50 carbon atoms. In 1974 the Nisshin Chemical Company in Japan began industrial production of CoQ and utilized tobacco-waste material from Southeast Asia. While supplies were still relatively limited, the breakthrough provided enough CoQ to make further medical trials of the nutrient possible. The Eisai Company, in Japan, took the bulk raw CoQ being manufactured by Nisshin and converted it into a pure pharmaceutical product available for clinical tests.

Then, in 1977, yet another revolution took place. The Japanese discovered a way of producing CoQ through fermentation and extraction from microorganisms—an inexpensive, self-replicating, endless production process. It was to become the standard for commercial CoQ production. It is interesting to note that this same method is used today to manufacture the majority of the antibiotics in use throughout the world at a fraction of previous costs. Many of the antibiotics bought under a recognizable western pharmaceutical company name in the United States are originally produced by chemical companies in Japan, bought in bulk, packaged, and then distributed under other names.

Shortly afterward the Kanegafuchi Chemical Company began putting out CoQ in unlimited amounts. The price of CoQ plummeted and within five years the cost had dropped from $1,000 a gram to less than $10!

Comments Karl Folkers, "As the production of CoQ_{10} by fermentation was increased, it became possible to explore clinical uses of CoQ_{10} without any limitation of supply. The passage of so many years of time between the chemical discovery of CoQ_{10} and the proof of efficacy to treat disease was controlled not by a lack of medical promise, but rather by a severe lack of supply to make possible clinical tests of utility. In biochemistry, CoQ_{10} is relatively old, but in medicine CoQ_{10} is relatively new."

How Is CoQ's Importance Viewed in the Scientific Community?

Soviet studies involving coenzyme Q have been quietly developing for the past two decades, and now it is considered an absolute priority in biomedical research. The Soviets have, in fact, created a new institute in the Ukrainian S.S.R. devoted entirely to CoQ research. It is the Quinone Research Institute in the city of Kiev. CoQ in the U.S.S.R. is produced for research purposes by the giant Soviet plant called Vitamin.

CoQ research has already played a key role in the creation of at least one Nobel laureate. Peter Mitchell received a Nobel Prize in 1978 for his research on the important new aspects of CoQ_{10} in mitochondrial energy transduction and his chemiosmotic hypothesis.

Like many brilliant discoveries leading to Nobel Prizes— the double helix of DNA is one example—Mitchell's inspiration came in a flash of insight. Mitchell put his thoughts on paper at about three A.M. on May 20, 1975, while suffering from insomnia. He modified his concepts of the reactions of CoQ_{10} to involve a cyclic system. This was the beginning of the evolution of ideas that have come to be known as the "Q-cycle"—a profound breakthrough in the understanding of how CoQ functions.

CoQ is now being made widely available in the United States where it is not yet classified as a prescription drug. It is sold over the counter as a food supplement. Meanwhile, the mass of scientific evidence to prove CoQ's benefits continues to boom in the United States.

CHAPTER 3

•

Revitalize and Boost
the Immune System:

With Emphasis on Cancer,
Infections, Chemotherapy, and Aging

Despite major research advances, infectious and allergic diseases remain high among the United States' great public health problems. Considered as a group, these diseases are the fifth leading cause of death, accounting for some one hundred thousand deaths a year.

According to the National Institute of Allergy and Infectious Diseases, patients with infectious diseases account for up to 30 percent of all visits to physicians' offices, and respiratory infections are the major cause of acute illness in the United States. Patients with allergies make at least 45 million visits each year at an estimated cost for care and medications totaling over one billion dollars. Infections and allergies are the primary responsibility of the immune system. A strong immune system is vital for warding off infections and combatting serious disease states.

Protection by the immune system involves millions of cells that defend vital organs and tissues, and which destroy invading organisms before they gain a foothold in the body. The immune system is a constant cellular battleground. And it is here that CoQ can play a crucial support role by strengthening and boosting the immune defenses, whether it's fighting off the common cold or battling cancer. Since the immune system is extremely complex, it is necessary to understand a little about its processes to help understand CoQ's role.

31

Getting to Know the Immune System

The most fundamental action of the immune system is in its ability to recognize anything foreign to the human body. Whether this is a bacterium floating in the blood stream, a virus hiding in tissue, or even a stray human cell drifting aimlessly around, the immune system will seek it out and destroy it.

The immune system is able to distinguish between "self" and "nonself," and it will act accordingly. It also has a memory for "faces," individual chemical markers that are displayed by foreign proteins. The immune intelligence remembers past invaders and reacts. Once a person has had mumps, the immune system instantly recognizes any further invasion attempt and swings into action, much faster and much more efficiently. That's why, for example, an individual who recovers from mumps will never get it again—unless the immune system and its surveillance techniques have suffered a major trauma in the meantime.

The chemical markers are called antigens. An antigen is any one of the millions of "nonself" molecules that can trigger an immune response. An antigen can be a virus, a bacterium, a fungus, a cancer cell or a parasite, or even a small molecular portion of one of these organisms.

Tissues and cells from another human individual—unless he or she is an identical twin—can also act as antigens, and are attacked. This is why in organ transplantation it is necessary to suppress the function of the immune system by using immunosuppressing drugs, like cyclophosphamide, cortisone, and cyclosporine.

The Immune Organs

The organs of the immune system are generally referred to as "lymphoid" organs because they are concerned with the development, growth, and deployment of white blood cells, most important of which are the lymphocytes. The lymphocytes are the mainstay of the defense network.

Immune system main bases include the bone marrow, the thymus, the lymph nodes, the liver, and the spleen. Other strategically positioned outposts are the tonsils, the appendix, and the clumps of lymphoid tissue in the small intestine known as Peyer's patches.

The lymphatic system itself is the line of supply throughout the immune network. The whole system is linked by lymph nodes, which are small bean-shaped structures spread throughout the body. Strings of lymph nodes can be found in the groin, abdomen, armpits, and neck. Lymph nodes act as depositories for cells of the immune system and also as centers for disposing of the remains of dead (or deceased) microorganisms.

This lifeline for the lymphatic system is a network of vessels similar to the blood vessels. These vessels constantly contain lymph, a clear fluid that acts as a carrier for the immune cells. Lymph also bathes the body's tissues and seeps backward and forward through the thin permeable walls of the smallest lymph vessels.

Immune Cells

Lymphocytes bear the brunt of the immune system work. They come in two main types, T cells and B cells.

The lymphocytes all originate in the bone marrow and are known as stem cells. Some cells migrate to the thymus, a multilobed organ that lies high behind the breastbone. Here they multiply and mature. These are the T cells that will go on to act as stimulant cells, motivating other immune cells when the body's immune competence is compromised. They are also responsible for suppressing the immune response once danger has passed.

B cells are those which mature in the bone marrow itself, or in immune organs other than the thymus. Their primary role during invasion by bacteria, for example, is to produce antibodies, specific chemical "bullets" that are deadly to the particular form of bacteria.

There are also natural killer cells; their name needs no explanation. Unlike B cells they work alone, need no stimulation from an antigen before they go into action, and endlessly patrol the body hunting down any type of foreign antigen. Normal healthy cells are resistant to natural killer cells, but most tumor cells and cells invaded by viruses are not—they display abnormalities which the killer cell spots. The natural killer cells play an important role in "immune surveillance" against cancer and other diseases, by hunting down any cells that develop abnormal characteristics.

Phagocytes are a special division of assassination and clean-up cells. The main cells with phagocytic actions are macrophages and monocytes. These are large cells that act as killer-scavengers—with the unique ability to engulf and digest foreign microorganisms and antigens. Macrophages ply their trade hidden in the tissues, while monocytes patrol by circulating in the blood.

Weapons of the Immune Cells

Most cells of the immune system use chemicals to attack invading organisms. The variety and amounts of chemical killers that can be produced by the cells of the immune system are immense. It has to be to meet the vast array of predators that can invade the human body. To effectively meet all these demands at the time of an infection, for example, the immune system would have to have stockpiled many different chemicals, each one coded for a specific virus or bacterium. But it doesn't. The immune system gets around this problem by manufacturing supplies of chemicals only when an invader is identified. The chemical weapons produced are specific to destroy that particular type of adversary.

Each foreign attacker displays a chemical marker on its surface. To neutralize the invader the defense cells produce an "antidote" to that chemical, and it fits the antigen's chemical marker receptor exactly, much like putting a key into a lock. Because there are millions of chemical variations, this has to be done on the spot when the invader is confronted.

When an invader is encountered, B cells spawn many new cells called plasma cells. Each one of these is a chemical factory in miniature that produces potent antibodies. These antibodies are of many varieties and are released into the bloodstream. Some of them will knock out other invaders they meet, and others will coat the surface of the invaders to make them more palatable and attractive to the phagocyte scavenger cells.

While this is going on the T cells will, in effect, oversee the ensuing conflict. T cells do not secrete antibodies, but their help is essential for antibody production because they can call in reinforcements of more B cells to the site of the action. When they stimulate B cells, the T cells are called helper cells. The T cells can also be powerful suppressors, and they will stop the production of deadly chemical weapons once the threat has been overcome. If it was not for the suppressor action of certain T cells, antibody production could run rampant and flood the body.

This only just touches on the immense variety of potential chemical weapons in the immune system's arsenal. These include complements, interferons, interleukins, and many others produced by various cells in the body. Only recently is the scientific community beginning to understand the interplay between these chemical weapons and the cells of the immune system.

Immune Response

Infections are the most common causes of human disease and are produced by bacteria, viruses, parasites, and fungi. They can range from relatively mild respiratory illnesses, such as the common cold, to dibilitating conditions like hepatitis and to life-threatening diseases such as meningitis and AIDS.

But to even get to infection stage, the invader must first find a chink in the body's defensive armor. The immune system has devised an entire network of defensive traps. It's no coincidence that the immune system deploys antibodies in the secretions of the respiratory and gastrointestinal tracts— the main gateways of entry and exit in the body. These guards are also found in high concentrations in other body fluids, like nasal secretions, tears, and saliva.

If bacteria have found an unprotected opening, in the skin for example, they then have to try to avoid the patrolling natural killer cells and the scavenger cells, which are unspecific in nature and will pounce on anything foreign.

Let's assume that the invading bacteria were so numerous that some managed to slip by the natural killers and the phagocytes. Now the invaders' problems are only just beginning.

Phagocytes will have already communicated to the T cells that foreign antigens are in the body. The T cells in turn will mobilize B cells to move in with their chemical weapons, and also bring in reserves of new phagocytes and natural killer cells with their individual arsenal of chemicals. This massive mobilization of cellular immune defenses, and production of munitions, requires extra energy (if you're playing bio-detective, you'll no doubt spot a CoQ link here).

If the infection is localized, say at the site of a flesh wound, inflammation and swelling will also occur, and these are both natural functions of the defense and healing processes. Once the infection has been overcome, the mopping up process begins. The dead on both sides are removed by the phago-cytes and other clean-up cells. They are then disposed of through the lymphatic system.

During this process some of the cells involved in the con-flict will become "memory" cells with the chemical "faces" of the invading bacteria permanently imprinted. The next time that this type of bacteria is encountered in the body, it will be instantly recognized before it is even able to gain a foot-hold. And the immune system would already be primed for combat. This memory is called secondary immune response, as opposed to primary immune response, which would result from a first meeting with an antigen.

Natural and Acquired Immunity

The human is born with relatively weak immune systems because much of the immune response is due to past experi-ence. The infant will have gained some natural immunity from its mother. It is passed through the placenta while the fetus is in the womb. More immune resistance is imparted after birth through the mother's milk. After that the immune system learns by experience.

Immunity can also be obtained through vaccines that will stimulate the immune response without developing into a full-blown disease state. Vaccines contain microorganisms, or parts of them, that have been altered enough for them to be impotent, yet able to create a reaction. Some vaccines are made from organisms that have been killed, others use organ-isms that have been "fixed" so that they can no longer pro-duce infection, for example, by multiplying. Some vaccines are made from live viruses that have been reproduced so many times in lab cultures that they lose their potency.

There can be drawbacks with vaccines. Microorganisms follow the rule of survival of the fittest, and consequently, when one strain is constantly being beaten back by the body's immune defenses, only the strongest will survive to repro-duce again.

Bacteria and viruses reproduce at such an astonishingly high rate that hundreds of new generations can live and die in a matter of hours. What genetic variation has taken thousands of years of evolution for the human body to make, can be achieved in a day or so for microbes. The strongest lines of bacteria will survive to create a new and more potent strain, usually with a slightly altered surface structure (antigen) to fool the immune system's memory. It's easy to see why in cases like influenza, which is particularly virulent, new vaccines have to be developed every year or so to keep up with their ever changing profiles. In cases of some infections and diseases it is necessary to have to keep updating the immune system's memory banks with new vaccines.

Immunodeficiency Disease

AIDS—or, acquired immunodeficiency syndrome—is a frightening disease. Immunodeficiencies are not new, but AIDS is different because its cause is not yet fully understood. And, at this point, there is no foolproof cure.

Some things that are known about AIDS will now make sense to you. AIDS is characterized by a very low level of helper T cells—the cells appointed to direct the mobilization of immune troops—while still displaying normal levels of the suppressor T cells. The AIDS virus invades the T cells and multiplies inside them, resulting in damage to the cells, causing immunodeficiency.

It should now be very obvious, because of the vast complexity of the immune system, that the lack of just one or more components can result in an immunodeficiency disease. These can be inherited, acquired through illness, or produced as an adverse side effect of certain drug treatments or various environmental factors, like radiation and toxic chemicals.

Some children are born with flaws in their B cell component and are unable to produce antibodies, leaving them vulnerable to infections. This condition can, however, be combatted with intramuscular injections of antibodies. Other children, whose thymuses are either missing or retarded, lack T cells. This can be corrected by treatment with thymus transplants or thymic extracts (thymic hormones). Very rarely, infants can be born with no immune factors whatsoever. These children, if they are to survive, have to spend their lives in germ-free rooms and "bubbles." There have been successes where these children have received bone marrow transplants from which the immature cells grow into functioning cells.

Advanced disease states, like cancer, can result in immuno-deficiencies as a result of the disease constantly taking its toll on the immune system. Some drugs used to fight disease states can also lower the immunity. Short-lived immuno-deficiencies can develop in the wake of common viral infections, including influenza, mononucleosis, and measles. Blood transfusions can also produce the same effect.

But to the apparently healthy individual, two factors can wreak havoc with the immune system. They are poor eating habits, resulting in malnutrition, and stress. Malnutrition is, even for our affluent society, a significant problem. And this is not usually the result of the lack of quantity of the foods we eat, but the lack of quality of the foods. Stress is a day-to-day problem for most people, the only difference is the varying degrees of stress we experience. Stress affects the brain, which we know today directs the various parts of the immune system. When high levels of stress are continually being experienced they can have the effect of depressing the immune system. This is where immune-boosting drugs may benefit certain stress-prone individuals.

An exciting area of pharmacology is the new immunopharmacology. It has flourished in the past decade with the result of substantial progress in the understanding of interactions of various components of the immune system. If immune response can be predictably boosted by drug intervention, then pharmacologic treatment of immunologic disorders could be feasible.

Providing you don't have any of the more serious acquired immunodeficiencies, you might consider yourself safe from a lack of immune response—but when we take into account the last two factors, stress and malnutrition, it leaves much of the population open to immunodeficiencies. This then is where CoQ can play a vital role, boosting a sagging immune system that may have become deficient in CoQ due to various factors including malnutrition and stress.

The CoQ Factor

Reviewing the mysteries of the immune system the following conclusions are apparent:

• An individual may feel drained of energy during such a period of full-blown immune invasion. The symptoms are increased temperature, weakness, tiredness, irritability, and listlessness.

• Fighting off illness and disease requires the activation of millions of cells, combined with the production of more cells and their individual chemical weapons. The essential extra energy for this doesn't just materialize, it has to come from increased bioenergetic process.

• Energy is produced at the cellular level, and Coenzyme Q_{10} is a crucial component in that energy production.

It should come as no surprise that most severe illness and disease states take hold as the body advances in age and the immune system begins to weaken. Is there a significant connection between age-related immune system deficiencies and the decline in the ability to supply internal CoQ_{10} with age? Many conclusions can be drawn as to the influences that might be considered to cause this natural and expected decline in the immune potential.

There is voluminous research to indicate that the immune system plays the single most significant role in how well, or how poorly, we age. Certainly we know that it is the one key factor in how efficiently we respond to illness and disease. Now there is also a growing body of work which indicates that CoQ plays a crucial role in the effectiveness of the immune system—and, therefore, in the way we age. CoQ and aging is discussed in Chapter 14.

If the human body doesn't have the necessary CoQ supplies needed to stimulate, reproduce, and maintain the cells of the immune system while under attack, the obvious end result is that the body will fall prey to a disease state.

Immune Boosting

George Bernard Shaw may have been closer to the truth than he might have suspected when he wrote a play called *The Doctor's Dilemma*, in 1906. One line in the play could have been an accurate prophecy of the direction in which medicine and research into the immune system was to turn eventually. It reads, "Nature has provided in the white corpuscles, as you call them . . . phagocytes as we call them . . . a natural means of devouring and destroying all disease germs. There is at bottom only one genuinely scientific treatment for all diseases, and that is to stimulate the phagocytes. Stimulate the phagocytes!"

The eminent man of letters had picked on only one component of the immune system—but the direction he chose was uncannily accurate. Throughout the past 30 or 40 years, science has indeed discovered that additional stimulation (or as scientists call it, modulation) of the immune system can be of paramount importance to the way the body fights illness and disease. Unfortunately, many of these stimulants are drugs, and their biggest drawbacks are that they are accompanied by various degrees of toxicity. For this reason they are not acceptable for practical clinical applications and are rarely turned to except as last resorts when a life-threatening immune deficiency is encountered.

Our work at the New England Institute on the relationship between CoQ and the host defense (or immune) system, was initiated with our first experiment performed on January 16, 1968. In this study we injected rats with newly available commercial CoQ_6 and measured the clearance of foreign matter (phagocytosis) from the blood circulation. This foreign material was removed twice as fast in CoQ_6 treated rats as compared with untreated animals. The significance of this experiment was that it displayed for the first time the power of CoQ to greatly enhance the process of phagocytosis, which is the removal of invading organisms from the blood circulation. The first publication of this breakthrough experiment took place in late 1968, and thus formed the foundation for all the following worldwide experimental work on CoQ and the immune system.

An important point to emphasize is that from the start of this early work, our own extensive toxicological studies, and those of other researchers in the field, revealed no abnormalities, side effects, or toxicity that would restrict the use of CoQ in humans. The immune stimulation, or modulation, that CoQ creates is produced by a mechanism totally unlike some of the immunodrugs in that it exhibits no problems resulting from toxicity.

The early work on CoQ_6 was then expanded to include CoQ_{10} as soon as supplies of Q_{10} became commercially available. With the utilization of CoQ_{10} a similar two-fold increase in the phagocytic rate was again observed. Then, in further experiments, we also established that CoQ_{10} increased the antibody levels in mice. As already explained the phagocytes and antibodies form a most powerful obstacle against invading organisms.

In antibody studies we found that mice treated with CoQ_{10} responded with a significantly higher level of antibody production. This level was more than twice as high as the level in untreated mice, with a high of 247 percent in the CoQ treated animals. Another significant point was that this immune boosting effect was achieved with only a single administration of CoQ. The results of these experiments, published in 1970 in the international biological journal *Experientia*, established for the first time the unique importance of CoQ for creating optimal activity in the immune system.

In a structure-activity relationship study published in *Chemical-Biological Interactions* in 1972, we evaluated activity of various members of the CoQ group using the rate of phagocytosis from the blood circulation of rats. Q_0 (CoQ devoid of the side chain) did not show any significant modification of phagocytic rate. CoQ_4, CoQ_6, and CoQ_7 produced a moderate effect, and CoQ_{10} produced the most pronounced effect. This study indicates that the activity of various CoQs increases relative to the length of the side chain.

Further confirmation of the beneficial effect of CoQ on the immune system was displayed in our experiments, which revealed its ability to reduce the number and size of chemically induced tumors in mice. It also increased the number of survivors. The tumors were purposely induced by the injection of dibenzpyrene, a chemical with very potent carcinogenic (cancer causing) effect. As an illustration of this chemical's dangerous potency, it is commonly present in tar and is a prime suspect for producing lung tumors in smokers. This type of chemically induced tumor is considered by scientists to most closely resemble naturally occurring tumors in humans.

By the 55th day after the administration of the carcinogen, 85 percent of the control (not treated with CoQ) group had developed tumors, and by day 69 it had extended to 100 percent. Meanwhile, among the CoQ treated mice only 25 percent displayed tumor growth at day 55; 65 percent at day 69; and only 77 percent at day 300!

Another parameter we looked at in the developing tumors in both groups was the tumor size, which was measured in square millimeters. At day 55 the control group displayed an average tumor size of 250 mm^2 (millimeters squared), compared to an average tumor size in the CoQ group of 95 mm^2.

By day 83 the control group size was 360 mm^2, and the CoQ group 170 mm^2. At day 97 the controls registered an average of 930 mm^2 compared to only 580 mm^2 in the CoQ treated group. Not only did fewer mice develop tumors in the CoQ group, but the tumors that did develop were significantly smaller.

Mortality was the third parameter we measured in this study. At day 83 5 percent of the control mice had died, with no fatalities in the CoQ camp. By day 111 50 percent of the controls were dead compared to only 15 percent of the CoQ mice. On day 132 all the control mice were dead, but even by day 300 80 percent of the CoQ benefited mice were still alive. This was an astounding life extending result, and especially when it is considered that the CoQ mice only received four injections of the nutrient, the last one being 21 days after the beginning of the experiment. It could be concluded that CoQ's lifesaving benefits had prevailed all the way through to at least the 300th day when the experiment was terminated.

Our studies using dibenzpyrene were published in the *Proceedings of the National Academy of Sciences* in 1973 and were presented at the 11th International Cancer Congress in Florence, Italy, in 1974. These findings, together with the 1970 publication, laid the foundation for fruitful research into CoQ as a nontoxic immunomodulating agent, and its ever increasing potential for practical clinical application.

Another significant breakthrough was made in a collaborative study together with Karl Folkers and his research group at the University of Texas. Together we discovered that deficiencies of CoQ would occur when an animal was infected with a virus. In the study it was found that a deficiency of CoQ was present in the spleens and white blood cells of mice infected with the virus. A specific leukemia virus, the Friend leukemia virus (also known as FLV), was used in these experiments. The reason for this was that it is very typical of viral infections, is highly predictable as a virus model, and has proven reliable quality. FLV infects various blood cells, including the important first line of defense, the macrophages. Organs of the immune system, like the spleen, have high concentrations of CoQ. The blood contains CoQ, and these levels can give a good general picture of CoQ throughout the body.

In this experiment the mice were split into two groups, one to act as a control group without being infected, and the second group to be infected with the FLV virus. The spleens of noninfected mice were found to display a CoQ deficiency of 36 percent. But 20 days after the introduction of the virus, the infected mice showed CoQ deficiencies of 62 percent. This difference clearly proved that a serious deficiency of CoQ was being produced after the virus had begun developing in the animal body. The blood of the control mice showed a deficiency of 24 percent, but in the infected group by day 20 it had grown to 36 percent. Table I illustrates the results of this experiment.

TABLE I

CoQ Deficiency in Mitochondria of Mice Infected with Friend Leukemia virus (FLV)

Sample	Group	Day after FLV Infection	Number of Mice	% Deficiency
Spleen	Control	Not infected	120	36
Spleen	FLV	5	40	44
Spleen	FLV	10	40	57
Spleen	FLV	20	40	62
Blood	Control	Not infected	120	24
Blood	FLV	5	40	30
Blood	FLV	10	40	31
Blood	FLV	20	40	36

It should be noted that some CoQ deficiency was observable in all the mice before the start of the experiment, but this became much more pronounced in the group of animals that were infected with the FLV virus. The deficiency of CoQ in the infected group worsened with the progression of the infection, and after day 20 when the deficiency in the spleen had reached 62 percent the mice began to die. This was a highly significant fact because this figure is very close to the predicted 75 percent deficiency of CoQ that is recognized as being incompatible with life in man. These results were published in the *International Journal for Vitamin and Nutrition Research* in 1975.

Another experiment was to prove the beneficial effects against a viral infection by boosting CoQ levels with supplements. In this study laboratory mice were infected again with FLV but when the mice received CoQ they showed a significantly lower mortality rate and less than half the total number of deaths than animals in the group that did not have the benefit of CoQ supplements. The mice that survived also exhibited an improvement in the clinical progression of the leukemia.

These experiments also showed that the FLV infection was accompanied by a general immunosuppression. But after CoQ supplements were administered to the mice, immunosuppression was significantly corrected. This immunosuppression was evaluated by the capability of the animals to produce antibodies. At the peak day of antibody production control animals (noninfected) produced over 160 units of antibodies. FLV infected mice produced only 40 units, or one fourth that of their noninfected counterparts. But when the FLV infected mice were treated with CoQ their production of antibodies increased to 80 units. These experiments revealed some striking relationships:

• The development of CoQ deficiencies in FLV infected mice.
• Reduced mortality in FLV infected mice treated with CoQ.
• The development of pronounced immunosuppression in FLV infected mice that was partially reversed by CoQ treatment.

It was a decisive indication of the indispensable role played by CoQ in maintaining optimal effectiveness of the immune system. Since human tumors, and especially leukemia, are manifested in the same manner as those of mice, it is to be expected that the human response would display similar beneficial effects after treatment with CoQ.

Malaria—the War We Thought Was Won

A next target for CoQ was to combat one of the world's most debilitating diseases, malaria. But why malaria? After the discovery of the malaria parasite and the identification of the Anopheles mosquito as the vehicle responsible for transmitting the parasite of this infection from person to person, new powerful antimalarial drugs were discovered. As a result this disease was almost wiped out: And, for some time it was, but now malaria is back with renewed vigor. Unfortunately the malaria parasite has grown resistant to drugs that were developed to combat it.

Quinine, a natural product from the bark of the cinchona bush, was the first effective antimalarial drug. At the beginning of World War II two new antimalarials became available. They were pamaquine (trade named Plasmochin) and quinacrine (Atabrine). A third generation of antimalarials produced chloroquine (Aralen), and chloroguanide (Paludrine). The most modern drugs are primaquine, sulfadiazine, and pyrimethamine.

The Anopheles mosquito, which was believed to have been killed off, found new ideal breeding grounds due to the "green revolution," organized to increase irrigation and food production in countries like India. It also became resistant to the powerful insecticides launched against it.

So, malaria has become a worldwide scourge once more, and, according to the World Health Organization, the problem of malaria has again reached epidemic proportions. According to a 1983 report by the Swiss Tropical Institute in Basel, malaria "affects more than 200 million people each year."

Obviously a new approach was needed to combat the disease of malaria. The approach selected by the World Health Organization and the U.S. Army Medical Service was immunotherapy. So, we set about testing CoQ's immune boosting abilities to aid in wiping out malaria altogether.

Using a new experimental malaria infection in mice, we showed in the laboratory that CoQ administration boosts the effectiveness of chloroquine, a drug of choice for the treatment of human malaria infections. CoQ treatment not only increased the number of mice surviving the infection but it also reduced the number of red blood cells infected by the malaria parasite.

Mice infected with malaria showed a mortality rate of 100 percent by the 21st day after malaria was introduced. At the same time the mortality rate of infected mice treated with chloroquine was 80 percent. But infected mice treated with CoQ and chloroquine showed a mortality rate of only 42 percent by day 21. In this experiment a single injection of CoQ was administered on the 3rd day after the malaria was induced. Clearly CoQ significantly improved the chemotherapeutic effect of chloroquine. But would CoQ work prophylactically to prevent malaria? This is a question of paramount importance for humans, and the next experiment answered it.

The study protocol mirrored the previous experiment, except for one vital difference: CoQ and chloroquine were administered 2 days before the infection. Twenty-one days after malaria was introduced mortality in the nontreated group was 98 percent, in the chloroquine treated group it was 80 percent, but the mortality rate in the CoQ-chloroquine pretreated group was only 55 percent. Another factor we established during these experiments was that the number of red blood cells infected by the malaria parasite in the CoQ-chloroquine group by day 7 after the infection was 80 percent less than the group treated by chloroquine alone.

The conclusion to be drawn from the human perspective is that CoQ and chloroquine together as a preventive measure clearly give protection against malaria; but if the disease is contracted, it is also obvious that if CoQ and chloroquine treatment is continued, this time therapeutically, an even greater beneficial response could be expected.

Now, research into antimalarial drugs is growing in the United States and throughout the world. Our studies showed for the first time that a new approach was possible for the treatment of malaria—via the modulation of the immune system—in combination with "classical" drug therapy.

In recognition of our research in this new approach to combatting malaria, we were invited to present our breakthrough research at the 3rd International Congress of Immunology in Sidney, Australia, in 1977, and later at the One Hundred Years of Malaria Research Symposium in Calcutta, India, in 1980.

Making Chemotherapeutic Drugs Safer with CoQ

Toxic drugs that are introduced into the body to kill off invaders or malfunctioning cells like leukemia and cancer work extremely well, but they also have unwanted side effects: they can knock out the immune protective responses at the same time.

In experiments where combining CoQ and chemotherapeutics, like cyclophosphamide (Cytoxan) or hydrocortisone, to battle induced leukemia in mice, the results were extremely optimistic. The most significant clinical symptom for the progression of leukemia is the dramatic enlargement of the spleen, caused partially by the build up of leukemia cells in the organ. For this reason the weight of the spleen is used as the most sensitive method of evaluating antileukemia drugs.

In the first experiment, mice that were infected with FLV

(Friend leukemia virus) showed an average spleen weight of 1.5 gm by day 20. In the group of animals treated with cyclophosphamide, the spleen weight averaged 1.4 gm (94 percent). In the group treated with single injections of CoQ and cyclophosphamide the spleen weights averaged 0.6 gm (45 percent).

In another experiment with the same protocol but using the chemotherapeutic agent hydrocortisone, we obtained the following results: the average spleen weight of FLV infected mice was 1.6 gm by day 20, mice treated with hydrocortisone displayed 0.9 gm (56 percent), and the group treated with hydrocortisone and CoQ showed 0.5 gm (34 percent). Clearly CoQ additions effectively retarded the clinical progression of the leukemia by boosting the effectiveness of the chemotherapeutic drugs.

One of the problems with many of the chemotherapeutic agents is that they produce strong immunosuppressive effects. For example, in organ transplantation in humans one of the clinically used drugs is Cytoxan, and its function is to depress the immune system to retard rejection of the organ. Cytoxan is also used to treat some forms of cancer, but at the expense of erasing the potential of the immune system.

In order to gauge immune suppression by Cytoxan we evaluated the ability of mice to produce antibodies. Normal mice showed 128 antibody units. A single injection of Cytoxan reduced the level to 80 units (63 percent). Now we looked at what action a single injection of CoQ would have on this immunosuppression and found that it resulted in the production of 113 units of antibodies (89 percent).

Adriamycin is another potent chemotherapeutic drug that has great value in the treatment of most forms of cancer. But the trade-off, once again, is the possibility of extreme toxic effects.

In a study, presented at the 12th International Congress of Chemotherapy, in Florence, Italy, during 1981, we evaluated the effect of Adriamycin on the immune system of mice. Adriamycin is an antibiotic of the anthracycline class and is regarded as the most important drug in cancer therapy. Our results showed that single Adriamycin administration produced a profound immunotoxic effect that results in extreme immunosuppression. This effect is associated with a significant reduction of the thymus and spleen weights, thus indicating further the involvement of the immune system. Charts A and B illustrate these effects.

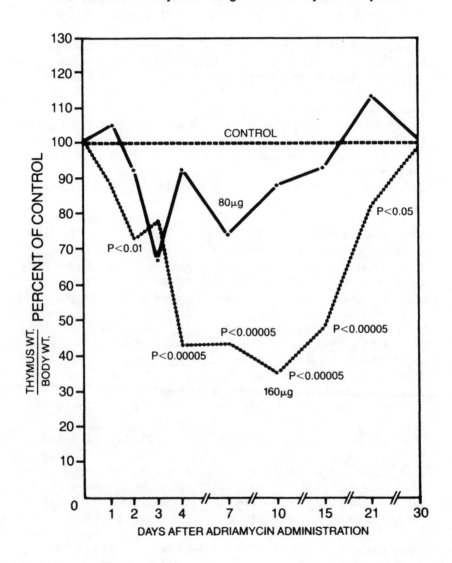

CHART A

Modification of Thymus Weight in Mice by Adriamycin

CHART B

Modification of Spleen Weight in Mice by Adriamycin

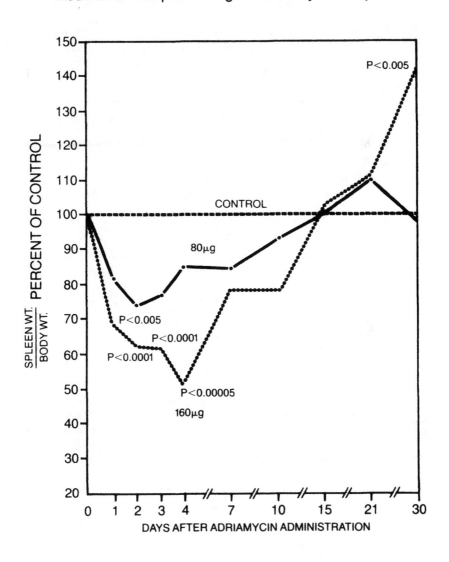

But administration of CoQ_{10} was able to produce a significant reversal of the Adriamycin immunosuppression. This was confirmed by comparing three groups of mice, one acting as a control, the second receiving Adriamycin only, and the third receiving Adriamycin and CoQ. When antigens were then introduced for testing immunoresponsiveness of the three groups, the control group reacted with a normal antibody response, the Adriamycin group showed depressed antibody response, but the CoQ_{10} treated animals showed a response close to that of the control group—thus reversing the immunosuppression originally caused by the Adriamycin. Chart C shows this result.

We concluded in our presentation, "Our studies indicate that Adriamycin, the potent immunotoxic agent, in its clinical use requires evaluation of the immune status of the patient. Furthermore, clinical use of Adriamycin in combination with Coenzyme Q_{10} in reducing cardiotoxicity should also take into consideration the altered state of the immune system by CoQ_{10} and its independent effect on the neoplastic process."

The results clearly indicated the beneficial role CoQ can play in boosting the immune system, while also protecting it against the unwanted side effects of chemotherapy. This led us to explore the possibilities of attempting to reproduce the same CoQ boosting effects in old animals whose immune systems might be naturally depressed.

Immunity and Aging

There is little doubt that the host defense system is subject to age-related changes occurring in animals and in man. These changes are characterized in general by a gradual decline of the activity in many compartments of the immune system. The decline forms the basis of a definitive relationship between old age and increased mortality due to infectious diseases and cancer in animals and man.

In our experiments we were able to determine without doubt that immune responses were naturally depressed in older mice. A single administration of CoQ to these animals showed an immediate reversal trend in this age-determined immune suppression. The antibody levels produced against a foreign antigen in young mice are almost 300 units. Older mice produce only about 130 units. CoQ treated elderly mice showed better than 240 units of antibodies.

CHART C

Suppression of Antibody Response (Hemolytic Units) by Adriamycin and Reversal by CoQ$_{10}$

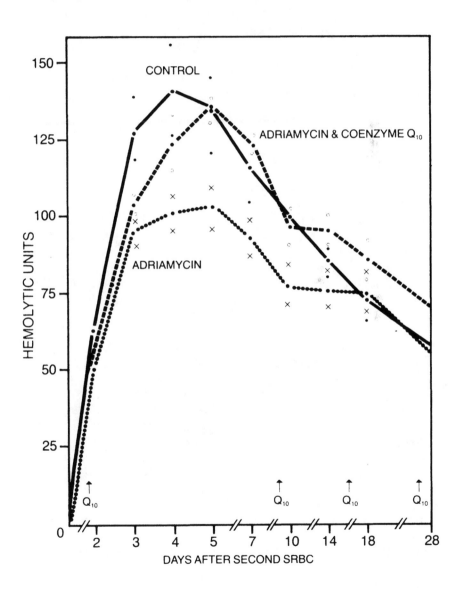

In another joint work with Karl Folkers's group, published in 1978, we looked at the relationship between the aging immune system and CoQ level. Old mice have only 20 percent of the normal CoQ level when compared to young mice.

Mortality in old untreated mice follows an expected age progression. We took very old mice, split them into two groups, and gave one group injections of CoQ. Some weeks after the start of the experiment all the untreated old mice had died of "natural" causes. At that time 40 percent of the treated mice were still alive. One mouse in the treated group died at week 82. Mean survival time in the untreated group was 20 weeks. The mean survival time of CoQ treated mice was more than 31 weeks, which is a 156 percent improvement.

Summary. Two logical conclusions were to be drawn from our important animal studies:

1. How much intracellular coenzyme Q there is available is apparently the limiting factor in the development of resistance in mice to aging, leukemia virus, other infections, and chemically induced tumors—the more CoQ available, the better the defense chances.
2. An increase in resistance can be created in mice that are subjected to infections, leukemia, tumors, and the "diseases" of aging by the addition of CoQ treatment—additional CoQ boosts resistance.

Our findings were presented to the scientific community in these words: "Experimental evidence indicates that the increased resistance in experimental animals conferred by coenzyme Q administration is mediated via stimulation of various parameters of the host defense system. This stimulation is not accompanied by significant cellular proliferation in the host defense system. Thus, we believe the stimulating effect is not a result of the activity of an increased number of cells but of a more efficient performance by existing cells."

What we were saying was that CoQ boosts the performance of immune system cells not by stimulating the production of more cells, but by inducing more energy, and thus increasing the immunocompetence, in the existing ones. They have more firepower without increasing in number. An interesting analogy might be equipping a small army with machine guns, instead of giving them hundreds of more soldiers armed with crossbows.

One of the most unwanted side effects of potent immunostimulating drugs is that they are so effective in producing an overbundance of new immunocells that the spleen becomes gorged with them, and expands like a balloon. In the human this is totally undesirable. This effect in itself is considered a form of toxicity of the immunodrugs.

In our immune system experiments, in order to prove a lack of this toxicity on the part of CoQ to the FDA, we removed normal size mouse spleens to provide data to FDA officials as proof that increased immunocompetence could be induced without the normally expected side effects from drugs that produced massive, bloated spleens.

CoQ's action had gone to the root of the problem: it was working at a molecular level by increasing the utilization of energy available to every single important cell in the immune system.

More Illuminating Research

Our pioneering work spurred on more scientists throughout the world to further probe the immune benefits of CoQ.

Referring to our research, Dr. Karl Folkers made the following observations:

There is considerable background information in the literature on Coenzyme Q_{10} and related quinones and the immune system. Extensive studies, which are possibly the most relevant to a specific effect of CoQ_{10} on the immune system, have been conducted by Emile Bliznakov and his co-workers. These studies of Bliznakov et al. began shortly before 1970 and continued to the early 80s. An account of this decade of research was given by Bliznakov at the Third International Symposium on the Biomedical and Clinical Aspects of Coenzyme Q in 1981. Some of the results are as follows: Various models were used to evaluate parameters of the immune system, including phagocytic rate, circulating antibody level, neoplasia, viral and parasitic infections. These models established the role of CoQ_{10} as an immunostimulating agent. The effect was enhanced when CoQ_{10} was administered in combination with other drugs.

During some pathological states, i.e., infection and ageing, organisms may develop a CoQ_{10} deficiency. All the results indicted that CoQ_{10} is an important component, probably at the mitochondrial level, for the optimal function of the immune system. The enhancement of the activity of the immune system by CoQ_{10} did not appear to result from hyperplastic alterations of the spleen, liver or other organs directly involved in the immune system response; it probably results from the increased activity of existing cells. It was concluded that CoQ_{10} is an appropriate candidate for clinical studies in disease states in which the immune system is not operating at optimal level.

Dr. Folkers is careful to emphasize the point that the effects of CoQ do not appear to stem from increased production of new immune cells, but from the increased potential of the already existing cells and their chemical defenses. The reader will no doubt recall the earlier point (and the lengths resorted to provide proof to the FDA), that it would be undesirable— and even potentially dangerous—to have massive production of immune fighters that would result in key immune system organs, like the spleen, being gorged with an excess of new immune cells.

This critical difference between the action of CoQ and other potential immune stimulants, is not only what makes CoQ so effective, but also completely safe.

Other scientists have not only tested CoQ_{10} but also other members of the coenzyme Q family. It's worth remembering at this point that even though an experiment may have utilized Q_7 or Q_8 in mice, whose own form of Q is CoQ_9, the injected CoQs must be made into Q_9 for it to work. The Q factor in humans is CoQ_{10}. Likewise, if CoQ_7 or CoQ_8 were utilized in human experiments, they would be transformed into CoQ_{10} to become effective.

Following our lead, new joint studies were instigated by researchers at the Yale University School of Medicine in New Haven, Connecticut, and the Sandoz Research Institute in Vienna, Austria. Here the enhanced resistance of mice to infections was tested utilizing CoQ_8. These results were published in 1978.

When mice were infected with the E. coli bacterium, Q_8 treated mice showed bacteria levels one hundred times lower than those of controls after 2 hours. After 10 hours the CoQ mice showed five hundred times fewer bacteria than their counterparts. This is the result of the activity of phagocytes, the killer-scavenger cells, thus confirming our results published in 1970. In Yale experiments, Q_8 significantly increased phagocytosis in CoQ treated mice, to four times the level in control animals. Daily injections of Q_8 maintained higher capacity of macrophages indefinitely.

The researchers reported: "Q_8 does offer a useful tool in the potentiation of nonspecific host resistance against a large spectrum of bacteria and is therefore of potential value in the chemotherapy of infectious diseases and cancer."

Further experiments involved testing the effects of CoQ_7 on the effectiveness of the immune system when artificially suppressed. The importance of this approach is obvious. We may often fall into an immune depressed state, say after a period of illness, when we are under great stress, or after surgery. It is when our immune systems are at their lowest ebbs that opportunistic organisms can rush in to take advantage of our lowered defenses.

Dr. J. Drews, from the Sandoz Research Institute in Vienna, utilized a potent immunosuppressant, the drug cyclophosphamide (Cytoxan), to reduce the number of granulocytes (one type of the leucocytes) in the blood systems of experimental mice. The effect of this drug was to induce an artificial lull in the immune defenses of the mice. This is the same drug we used in our experiments, and referred to earlier.

As a first phase to the study, the mice were injected with the suppressing agent. A normal response to the drug would be an immediate drop in granulocytes as they were killed off. Then a gradual rise in the number of these immune system warriors would be observed as the immune system reacted and rebuilt the granulocyte defenses.

The immune compromised animals were divided into two groups and half of them then received a shot of CoQ_7, 3 days after the start of the experiment. It soon became very obvious that the mice receiving CoQ began to rebuild their immune defenses much faster than those without the benefit of CoQ. Chart D illustrates this response.

The mice were then injected with lethal dosages of four virulent organisms—Pseudomonas aeruginosa, E. Coli, Klebsiella pneumoniae, and Candida albicans—all of which will cause massive infections in humans and can lead to death if the immune system is in a suppressed state. It is organisms of

CHART D

Immune Response following Suppression and after Addition of CoQ7

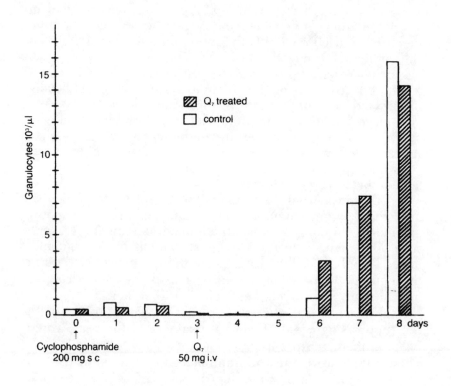

this type that can cause life-threatening conditions, such as pneumonia.

All the mice were injected with cyclophosphamide immunosuppressant, and then exposed to the deadly organisms. But some batches of mice had the benefit of first being pretreated with CoQ_7 before the organisms were introduced.

Table II shows the different results of the mice with injections of CoQ_7 and those that received only a saline (salt) solution to act as controls.

TABLE II

Protective Effects of Q_7 against Experimental Infections with Opportunistic Organisms

Infection	Survivors by Day 15*		Average Survivors	
	Control	Q_7 treated	Control	Q_7 treated
Pseudomas aeruginosa	0	12	2	10.4
E. coli	7	20	6.6	15.0
Candida albicans	4	11	4.4	12.1
Klebsiella pneumoniae	0	2	3.5	6.1

*Termination of experiment.

Chart E clearly illustrates the lethal effect the organism pseudomonas had on the control group as compared to those treated with CoQ_7.

Another important aspect of immune defense response was assessed by measuring the levels of phagocytosis in the bloodstreams of mice. Groups of ten mice were given injections of either CoQ_7, or saline solutions (to act as a control).

The numbers of macrophages (killer-scavenger cells) were then measured by the amounts of erythrocytes (specially labeled cells) they were able to ingest and consume. The boost in macrophages after CoQ_7 treatment is evident in the following table (Table III).

CHART E

Survival Rate of Granulocytopenic Mice after Pseudomonas infection

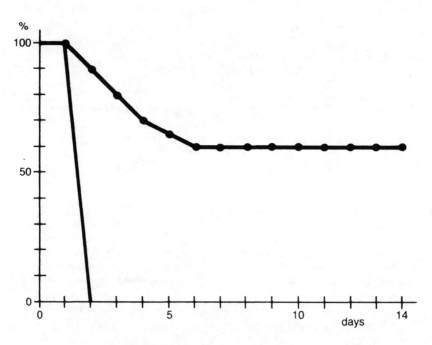

Straight line indicates control group.
Dotted line indicates CoQ_7 treated animals.

TABLE III

Treatment	Macrophage Activity
Saline (control)	443
Ubiquinone Q_7	1713

It is obvious from these animal studies that coenzyme Q can play a powerful role in the protection and stimulation of the immune defense system. This study confirms our 1970 findings.

What follows is a synopsis of selected studies involving the work of other researchers worldwide with coenzyme Q and the immune system.

• Institute of Immunological Science, Hokkaido University, Japan. Mice tested for the boosting of immune system macrophages (killer-scavenger cells) by coenzymes Q. Control tests show average differential cell count of macrophages to be 83.2. First day of CoQ_7 treatment counts jump to 94.3 and by the 3rd day, 95.7.

Researchers report: "In this study we found that ubiquinones and their related compounds enhanced the various functions of mouse peritoneal macrophages and that structural requirements might exist in the expression or augmentation of macrophage activation. Consequently, ubiquinones and their related compounds could be considered to stimulate the host defense mechanisms against microorganisms and neoplastic cells via macrophage activation."

• Department of Internal Medicine, Medical School, Osaka University, Japan. Coenzyme Q acids boost immune response. All the quinonyl acids (acids related to coenzyme Qs) tested on mice enhanced the immune response two to seven times, 5 weeks after immunization. Individually, high doses of CoQ_7 and CoQ_2 derivatives enhanced the immune response to a level two to three times that of the control animals.

Researchers report: "All the compounds tested in this study enhanced the immune response about two to seven times as much as that of the control group."

• National Cancer Center Hospital, Tokyo, Japan. Restoring immune functions in cancer-stricken mice with BCG (a powerful, but toxic, immune system booster) and CoQ_{10}. Mice with induced cancer tumors were treated with BCG and then with CoQ_{10}. Immune function was slightly increased with BCG alone. It was greatly enhanced by the additional treatment of CoQ.

Researchers report: "These results show that Coenzyme Q_{10} enhances the immunorestoration with BCG in tumor-bearing mice."

The Vitamin E and Selenium Connection

Vitamin E has been promoted for its role in healing and cell protection. There's no doubt about E's role as an essential vitamin, but some researchers have puzzled over the mechanics of its curious actions within the immune system. A typical, often quoted research reaction to vitamin E's beneficial abilities is: "The mechanism of increased humoral immunity and protection by vitamin E is not yet clear." Now a clue to explain the possible secret of vitamin E's powers has come to light—its role in enhancing increased production of CoQ.

There's a growing body of research to show that the vitamin's effect on the immune system is not in its own specific action, but in its ability to be used as building material in the production of coenzyme Q.

Studies by Dr. Rollin H. Heinzerling, in the Department of Microbiology at Colorado State University, confirmed that vitamin E can protect mice against infections. In a series of experiments, doses of vitamin E were administered to four groups of 35 mice, some immunized and others nonimmunized against a lethal dose of the microorganism Diplococcus pneumoniae. In nonimmunized mice the supplemental vitamin E raised their survival rate from 20 to 80 percent when compared to control animals. In the immunized mice, the vitamin treated group also showed four times more phagocytic activity than untreated immunized controls.

Dr. Heinzerling's comments on how he believes vitamin E achieved this effect make intriguing reading: "A similar biphasic phagocytic effect was observed by Bliznakov and Adler in studying the effect of Coenzyme Q_{10} on phagocytosis . . . The similarity of action of ubiquinones (in the Bliznakov experiments) and of vitamin E in ours suggests a possible common mode of action.

"In some very recent experiments (unpublished data) we have observed an increased ubiquinone synthesis stimulated by vitamin E. One possible mode of action of vitamin E could be an increased ubiquinone synthesis leading to a more efficient electron transport and metabolism in phagocytic and immunocompetent cells. This mode of action would also explain why vitamin E acts, or [is] purported to act, on so many different cells or cellular functions."

Further confirmation of the use of vitamin E to build coenzyme Q is provided by scientists at the A. V. Palladin Institute of Biochemistry, Academy of Sciences, in Kiev, in the U.S.S.R. Soviet scientist Dr. H. V. Donchenko compared vitamin E and vitamin A, and found that only vitamin E would boost CoQ biosynthesis. In studies of rats he discovered that doses of vitamin E would increase the content of CoQ in the liver by 30.2 percent and in the kidneys by 12.8 percent. The same scientists also found that in rats suffering from a vitamin E deficiency, the level of CoQ in the liver was decreased by 16 percent.

Dr. Donchenko confirms, "The data obtained is evidence for a linkage between ubiquinone and vitamin E content in an organism. Such a dependence is not found for vitamin A."

The role played by selenium, a trace mineral, in human health is highly controversial. Selenium has come from being an element considered 10 or 15 years ago as detrimental to human health, to being accepted today as one of the basic nutrients essential for maintenance of optimal health. Twenty years ago selenium was suspected of being a cancer-causing agent occurring naturally in tap water. Today it is being viewed as a trace mineral with anticancer activity. It has already been used therapeutically by the cattle industry to treat common bovine muscular diseases.

Two of the pioneers in selenium research, D. V. Frost and R. Van Poucke, wrote in a review published in 1973, "biosynthesis of the ubiquinones depends on the nutrient adequacy of selenium. There seems to be no doubt that selenium is needed for ubiquinone production. Addition of selenite to rations not deficient in selenium increased tissue levels of ubiquinones." From this research perspective it is clear that the effect of selenium as an anticancer agent is closely linked to its importance in the production of cancer-fighting CoQ.

Findings like these and the rationale that vitamin E, or selenium, boost CoQ's biosynthesis provide further reinforcement of CoQ's beneficial powers.

Human Immune Power

As we learn more about CoQ and its action of protecting and boosting the immune system through bioenergetics, it becomes evident that many of us are experiencing our own internal energy crisis.

As with all beneficial drugs that are eventually made available to the public, years of extensive and extremely detailed tests with animals have to be performed. This is an essential safety factor required by the FDA.

It has been explained exactly where CoQ stands with the FDA. The criteria have been satisfied that CoQ produces absolutely no toxic effects in animal models. Today the FDA has introduced new guidelines for new experimental drugs which require that before human trials can begin, the drug has to be proven, without doubt, that it performs a beneficial effect in animal studies.

It is clear that CoQ does meet all the stringent requirements of the FDA. Experiments involving CoQ's effect on the immune system are now cleared for human experimentation. An optimistic start has now been made on studies of CoQ and its relationship to the human immune system.

The following recent study offers new insights into the beneficial potential of CoQ supplements to increase immune power.

One antibody produced by the cells of the immune system is immunoglobulin (or antibody) G—known as IgG, for short. IgG is the major antibody in the blood. It is one of the antibodies that coats microorganisms to make them more palatable and speed their uptake by the scavenger immune cells. It is therefore one of the key players in the immune response. During studies on the effects of CoQ in the treatment of patients in a variety of disease states, an exciting discovery was made: there was a distinct increase in the levels of immunoglobulin G. Eight patients were involved in this particular study conducted by Dr. Karl Folkers at the Institute for Biomedical Research at the University of Texas. Four of them had cardiovascular disease, one had a form of diabetes, and three had cancer. All the patients received oral dosages of 60 mg of CoQ per day, three capsules containing 20 mg each.

Previous studies of IgG in blood showed that normal levels of immunoglobulin G anywhere between 700 and 1,400 mg/dl could be expected. Obviously this disparity in readings may depend very much on the individual. Take the figure of 900 on the scale; while this might be within perfectly normal range for one individual, it may represent a serious deficiency for another. Taking that into account, here are some of the results of this study.

Boosts of IgG were observed in two of the patients by day 35 of CoQ therapy. Four other patients exhibited significant increases by the 64th day, and one patient by day 97. The only patient who did not display any IgG effect was boosted to 100 mg of CoQ a day, and his IgG did respond with a significant rise by day 132.

One patient, a 69-year-old female with cancer of the breast, showed a rise from 940 mg/dl of immunoglobulin at the start, to 1437 after 90 days of CoQ administration.

Another patient, a 66-year-old male with cardiac failure, jumped from 1053 to 1258; a 65-year-old male with diabetes, from 1100 to 1305; and the IgG levels of a 75-year-old male with cancer of the lung went from 843 to 1028.

A report of this study concluded that "an increase in levels of IgG from lower to higher levels" could indicate a reduction in immunodeficiency, and "an increase in immunocompetence," simply by the addition of CoQ.

The Future of CoQ and Immunity

The immune system is becoming one of the most important topics of conversation today when people talk about ill health, disease states, and cancer. And there is little doubt that in the very near future the immune system will be recognized as the first line of defense when it comes to combatting deadly diseases like cancer.

Recent developments in medical pharmacology have focused on attacking an invader directly, rather than finding the root cause and directing therapy from there. Present-day reasoning tends to mirror the old adage "kill or cure." Unfortunately this approach most often results in temporary improvements rather than a permanent cure.

It is because of this mentality in research that CoQ's potential has been very much overlooked in the field of immunity. And it may be that treatment of the entire human immune system with the nutrient CoQ could alleviate the necessity to develop individual chemical medications aimed specifically at diseased cells and tumors. Alternatively, low doses of drugs, with less consequent toxicity, in conjunction with CoQ will produce an optimal effect.

So far, research into CoQ and the human immune system has taken a back seat to the more easily demonstrable effects of CoQ in, for example, heart disease. It's only natural that the attention of the scientific community and also of the public, should be drawn to disease states where the reduction of symptoms are easier to illustrate and report on. It is indeed easier to understand how increasing the bioenergetics of cells in the heart can alleviate and prevent heart problems, but it takes a little more to convince people that boosting the energy potential of cells in the immune system can possibly cure and prevent cancer.

Our research with animal models, and the studies of other scientists, have proved conclusively that CoQ can produce a profoundly beneficial effect on the immune system—the defense system that is already under strain and attack by infections and disease states. And it is equally clear that CoQ can boost the potential of helpful chemotherapeutic drugs by protecting against their unwanted toxic effects.

The Phase I trials we performed jointly in the mid-seventies with clinicians at the Yale Medical School, in New Haven, Connecticut, involving terminal cancer patients, have proved that CoQ displays no toxic side effects whatsoever. These clinical studies, under the auspices of the FDA, show that CoQ is much safer than many drugs presently on the market.

It also follows that CoQ supplements to the immune system should do nothing but exert a safe and powerfully prophylactic effect against the onset of deadly disease states. Overall, the action of CoQ on the immune system is profound, it promotes bioenergetic processes in the human immune cells that may prove to be the key to curing many of the diseases that ail us, and the ravages of old age.

CHAPTER 4

•

The Heart Link

Heart disease is the leading cause of death in the United States. Taken together, all cardiovascular, lung, and blood diseases accounted for some 1,200,000 deaths a year in the early 1980s—or 56 percent of all deaths. They are also a heavy financial drain on the economy, accounting for in excess of $122 billion, or 25 percent of the total economic cost of illness and premature death.

The National Heart, Lung, and Blood Institute compiled the following statistics:

• Cardiovascular diseases cause one out of every two deaths.
• Cardiovascular diseases cause almost 1 million deaths each year:
    —76 percent due to atherosclerosis
    —550,000 due to coronary heart disease
    —160,000 due to cerebrovascular diseases
• Cerebrovascular disease is the third leading cause of death.
• Heart disease, hypertension, and cerebrovascular diseases rank among the ten leading chronic conditions causing limitation of activity.
• States in Appalachia have the highest death rates for coronary heart disease and are experiencing the least decline in rates.

However, there are encouraging new statistics:

• States in the Southeast have the highest death rates from cerebrovascular disease, but are experiencing the steepest decline in rates.

• In 1983, the death rate for coronary heart disease was 60 percent of what it was in 1963.

• Between the early sixties and the early eighties, the death rate for all cardiovascular diseases declined much more rapidly than did the rate for all other causes of death.

• By the early eighties, heart disease no longer was the leading cause of death under age 65.

• The drop in cardiovascular disease deaths since 1948 has been so significant that by the early eighties there were 690,000 fewer deaths a year from these diseases than would have occurred had the death rate not declined.

• Among 26 industrialized countries, the United States
—Has the steepest decline in cardiovascular mortality in middle-aged men.
—Has the steepest decline in mortality from coronary heart disease in men and women ages 35 to 74 years.

The war against cardiovascular disease is far from over. But we now have a powerful new ally—Coenzyme Q_{10}.

Heart Mechanics

The heart is the most vital of our life-sustaining organs. Yet, paradoxically, it could be considered the simplest. It is, in mechanical terms, a very basic pump. It doesn't have any independent internal moving parts like impellers or pistons to wear out or break down.

The mechanics of the heart is simply like a squeeze bag. Compared to some of the other organs the heart is primitive elegance. While the brain is performing its constant mental gymnastics with electrical and chemical impulses running through myriads of neurons, dendrons, and synapses, the heart is efficiently beating. While the biological factory of the liver is performing biochemical alchemy at a rate that would stagger a Nobel laureate, and the kidneys are purifying and filtering, the heart just keeps up its simple pumping action. But without an efficient heart and cardiovascular system, the other more complex organs are doomed to failure.

From the biomechanical viewpoint this cardiac pump is a clever integration of muscles that expand and contract in a strictly regimented sequence to pump blood. The only hint of real sophistication in this four-chambered muscular sack is the one-way valves that stop the blood flowing backward once it has been pumped from one compartment to another.

Each day the healthy heart beats one hundred thousand times and pumps 4,300 gallons of blood—or 1.5 million gallons a year. Without interruption it accepts returned spent blood, depleted of oxygen and high in carbon dioxide, on one side, blasts it into the lungs for a rejuvenating boost of oxygen, takes it back and forces it out on the other side, back into circulation throughout the entire body. It is the single force of the heart's pumping action that keeps the blood circulating through every tissue of the body.

This process goes on nonstop throughout an entire lifetime. And yet the vital organ is only a large mass of muscle fiber. Consider other muscle structures, like the ones that raise and lower the forearm. Try sitting down and doing continuous arm lifts for an entire day, or even just a few hours, and see how much the muscles complain and object with pain. The heart doesn't usually let out a whimper on its lifelong odyssey of pumping.

There are clinically three groups of heart diseases that are important from the CoQ standpoint:

1. *Congestive heart failure* is a clinical syndrome in which the heart fails to maintain an adequate output resulting in diminished blood flow to the tissues and congestion in the lungs or in the blood circulation.

2. *Myocardial ischemic disorder* is a syndrome in which the blood supply to the heart muscle is diminished, usually resulting from coronary artery disease (chronic artereosclerosis) or myocardial infarction (abrupt reduction of coronary blood flow).

3. *Angina (pectoris)* is a special class of myocardial ischemic disorder that results from various kinds of stress, including psychosomatic and physical.

Many drugs are used to alleviate these cardiac disease states but no permanent cure is available.

Like every other muscle in the body, the heart needs essential nutrients to supply it with the energy needed for its constant miracle of endurance performance. This is why the highest concentrations of coenzyme Q in the human body are to be found in cardiac muscle.

The CoQ-Cardiac Pathway

In 1957, some time after the role of CoQ had been recognized as essential for the natural well-being of healthy cells, biomedical scientist Dr. Karl Folkers had a suspicion that CoQ could also play an important role in the functioning of the heart. Dr. Folkers had also discovered the importance of vitamin B_6 and had been the first to synthesize this essential nutrient. It was to be years before the profound importance of B_6, a landmark in human nutrition, was fully appreciated.

The scientist suspected that CoQ existed naturally in the human heart and was a unique and valuable nutrient to the heart's energy source. The name "bioenergetics" was later coined to describe the union of energy and life at the cellular level. Folkers believed CoQ was vital to the bioenergetic process.

Over 25 years later the theories concerning CoQ's necessity to the heart have been scientifically proven beyond doubt. And today Dr. Folkers has come to another dramatic conclusion: diseases of the heart may actually be caused by a lack of vital CoQ.

The man recognized as the father of CoQ research in the United States, states categorically, "Today, I am fully satisfied to know that CoQ_{10} is truly present in mitochondrial bioenergetics, and I am fully content to believe that a deficiency of CoQ_{10} may be a disease to be treated by oral administration." He adds, "I believe it is quite possible that cardiovascular disease may be very significantly caused by a deficiency of CoQ_{10}."

These are dramatic words when one considers that cardiac failure and its ancillary disease states are the single biggest terminators of life in our present society. Here is a biomedical scientist suggesting that we might be able to prevent the nation's number one killer by the simple oral supplementation of a natural nutrient to our diets.

The same nutrient might also act as a treatment for cardiac disease victims by strengthening the heart's bioenergetic processes and prolonging its potential life span and capacity for further work.

First Steps in Research

In the early days of research into CoQ's link with the heart, Dr. Folkers and his fellow researchers obtained seven human hearts from the autopsy table. These organs were carefully dissected and samples were taken for further examination in the laboratory. Using newly developed biochemical methods, the samples were analyzed and, through extraction techniques, a yield of chemically pure crystalline CoQ_{10} was isolated from the tissues. This simple first step was to have far-reaching consequences for the entire future of CoQ research—and the understanding of one of the most essential biochemical strength processes in the human heart.

The Folkers data gave proof that CoQ exists naturally in the human heart. Its exact function at that time was unknown, but Dr. Folkers again followed his own suspicions that CoQ was crucial to the heart's bioenergetics. To fit the next piece into the puzzle, the researchers looked for a correlation between levels of CoQ in the diseased heart and CoQ in the healthy heart. They were not to be disappointed.

A good starting point to seek a nutrient in the body is in the blood. The circulatory system supplies the entire body with its essential nutrients derived from the nutrients we ingest as foods. Analyzing blood samples is a relatively noninvasive method of gauging what's occurring in internal systems and organs.

At this point in the research it would not have been considered prudent, or even necessary, to attempt to collect samples of living human cardiac tissue, although studies on animal hearts were beginning to show the critical importance of CoQ, and the unfortunate end results of the lack of it.

Dr. Folkers, together with Japanese co-worker Tatsuo Watanabe, collected blood samples from a total of one hundred patients who were all diagnosed as suffering from various states of cardiac disease, and compared them to samples obtained from a control group of the general population without diagnosed heart problems.

In technical terms, what they discovered was that the cardiac patients displayed a mean specific activity of Coenzyme Q_{10} in their blood, which was computed at the figure of 3.06. The healthy control group's blood tests showed a CoQ reading of 4.20. In simplified terms, the cardiac group was functioning with blood levels of CoQ that were less than

three-quarters those of the healthier subjects. In scientific
jargon the CoQ levels for the cardiac victims were "significantly lower."

If blood levels showed a disparity in the amount of CoQ
between healthy and diseased subjects, what would the actual heart reveal? The Folkers team went on to obtain cardiac
biopsies from surgery performed by heart specialist Dr. Den-
ton Cooley. Again, the search for CoQ produced more dramatic results. There was a total of 132 biopsies made available
that covered a wide spectrum of thirteen different categories of heart disease. Laboraory analysis showed an undeniable CoQ connection. A massive 75 percent of the cardiac
patients showed varying but significant deficiencies of CoQ in
their heart tissue. This figure of 75 percent will take on major
significance.

In Japan, clinical studies on the effects of CoQ in populations of cardiac patients were progressing at a frenetic pace.
An important commercial reason was responsible for this
surge in interest—simple supply and demand, the Japanese had
discovered the pharmaceutical method to mass produce CoQ.

Later in his research, Dr. Folkers was to review studies
that had been performed in Japan. He examined no less
than 25 scientific papers that involved clinical reports from
110 physicians in 41 Japanese medical institutions for a period
of 9 years prior to 1976. All the studies, involving thousands
of patients, were on the beneficial effects of administering
CoQ to patients with congestive heart failure.

From almost a decade of the most thorough clinical research, which included two large double-blind trials, Dr.
Folkers was able to draw one important conclusion—beneficial
therapeutic effects were reported in at least 70 percent of
heart disease victims.

The tie-in with Dr. Folkers's earlier findings from diseased
heart tissue biopsies was undeniable. His experiments had
revealed CoQ deficiencies in three-quarters of cardiac victims. Like a mirror image from across the globe, the Japanese research teams were reporting dramatic benefits from
CoQ supplementation in three-quarters of their heart disease
patients.

Every available heart function test showed significant improvement in cardiac performance, and—most important to
the scientific community—the results were not just subjective but they were highly "significant" and clinically repeat-

able. CoQ was no longer a bewildering enigma. Dr. Folkers reported on the findings, "Such clinical benefits from treatment with CoQ_{10} appears to be due to correction of deficiencies and improvement of bioenergetics."

Between 1976 and 1980, 4 million cardiac patients were treated with CoQ in Japan. In 1979 alone about 1.5 million victims of heart disease received CoQ. Today the number of Japanese taking CoQ under medical supervision, as a prescription drug, for heart problems is estimated at well over 10 million.

In the United States, researchers like Dr. Folkers are actively promoting the benefits of CoQ through their continued studies. American and European pharmaceutical companies are making unprecedented reappraisals of the commercial and health benefits of CoQ, especially for medicinal use under strict conditions that satisfy the various medical governing bodies.

At the 4th International Symposium on coenzyme Q in 1983, Dr. Fritz Zilliken of the Department of Physiological Chemistry at the University of Bonn, in Germany, gave a thought-provoking reminder of the health potentials of CoQ. He told an audience of medical scientists, "It has taken almost 30 years after the discovery and synthesis of vitamin B_6 by Karl Folkers until its absolute requirement for men—say children—has been discovered by accident. Similar statements could be made for the action mechanisms of Aspirin and penicillin!"

A public awareness of the undoubtable benefits of CoQ may help to speed up this process, not only with conditions of the heart, but also with the immune system and the numerous other disease states that benefit from CoQ.

The proof of CoQ effectiveness in heart disease is impressive. Many tests have shown not just dramatic improvements, but possibilities of protecting the heart phrophylactically. The only way to appreciate the benefits of CoQ is to review these encouraging studies.

CHAPTER 5

•

Cardiac Wonders

One issue that became of major significance during the very earliest stages of research into CoQ's role in heart tissue was the noticeable decrease of the coenzyme in diseased states. This significant clue may have drifted into oblivion had the lack of CoQ been nothing more than a deleterious effect of the disease process. The necessary uptake of nutrients is usually expected to suffer when a disease takes hold, but with CoQ there was a difference.

Deficiencies of CoQ were found only in troubled hearts. Those that were healthy and functioning well were observed to have an adequate amount of CoQ in the tissue. What made this finding so special was that when supplemental CoQ was introduced into the ailing heart it began to take on renewed vigor.

The obvious conclusion had to be drawn that CoQ was not only necessary for the proper functioning of the heart, but when levels of CoQ began to drop, a disease state could be expected to take over, or have already done so.

But reintroduce CoQ and boost its levels back to normal, and something very important begins to happen: tissues that had been affected—possibly through lack of energy, and therefore incapable of fighting off the problem—take on a healthier glow, appear to be revived by an influx of energy, and take an aggressive stance against the disease.

For several years it has been known that CoQ is essential to the bioenergetics of all cells at the mitochondria level. Some of the hardest working cells in the human body are in muscle tissue and consequently need a good supply of energy.

• It's a fact that the heart is one of the strongest and hardest-worked muscles in the human body, and because of

72

its constant performance among the muscular systems, it obviously needs an abundance of energy.

• It's a fact that more CoQ is found in heart tissue than in any other muscle in the body.

• It's also a fact that as our own natural ability to maintain sufficient CoQ levels in our body declines, so can CoQ levels in the heart, and eventually the heart's overall performance must be affected.

The decline of CoQ appears to occur with age, leaving the heart with less than peak energy levels at a time when it might be most vulnerable to the diseases of aging.

We've already discussed how and why we can accumulate CoQ_{10} naturally in our body from foods that contain various kinds of CoQ, and the fact that the ability to perform the chemical changes necessary to produce CoQ declines with age. Unfortunately it is impossible to predict when or where the production cutoff point is. We do know that some people age "better" than others.

Why one individual has a better ability to weather the rigors of life rather than another, may eventually be narrowed down to the point in biological time when the body no longer has the ability to maintain sufficient levels of CoQ. The immune system and the heart both depend heavily on adequate supplies of CoQ, and they are both usually the first to suffer from the breakdowns of old age. The octogenarian who has hardly ever suffered anything more than an occasional cold or flu is more likely to have a body that's still maintaining optimum levels of CoQ. The 40-year-old who has high blood pressure and suffers his first coronary is more likely to exhibit a distinct deficiency of CoQ.

The most vexing problem is to be able to predict when the autonomic switch controlling the production of CoQ_{10} from the lower Qs turns itself off. Indeed, we suspect that it must do so at some stage because of the lack of CoQ in aging and diseased systems. There may be many more years of research before we can pinpoint the reason for this biological phenomenon, but until then we can simply introduce additional supplements of CoQ into the body.

CoQ Does Not Act Like a Drug

It is important to remember when reviewing CoQ studies that the nutrient does not have the same, almost instantaneous, action as a pharmaceutical drug. The coenzyme's action is vitamin-like. Drugs are expected to exhibit their effects in minutes, hours, or days, and the action has to be renewed with further dosages. Vitamins and nutrients, such as CoQ, take days and often weeks for absorption and utilization. There's a very sensible reason for the slowness of this action.

A vitamin's role is to affect biological systems at a molecular level, which will in turn create an eventual overall effect. Vitamin A, for example, can be toxic in high dosages, so the body protects from this happening by only absorbing it in small amounts. Water soluble vitamins, such as B, are utilized immediately and the body discards what it doesn't need at that time so that toxic levels are never allowed to build up. Vitamins like the A vitamins, which are fat soluble, can be stored harmlessly in fatty tissues and are mobilized as needed to replenish cellular levels.

CoQ is fat soluble, but it is not fully understood whether it can therefore be put into storage and pulled out when available supplies run low. When a deficiency of a fat soluble vitamin occurs, it is generally the result of existing stored supplies being gradually exhausted over a long period of time. To correct a vitamin deficiency the body begins to rebuild its stores while utilizing some of the new supplies to make up the deficit that exists in the tissues. But just as a vitamin deficiency takes a long period to develop, so does correcting the problem and bringing the biological chemical equations back into balance.

A similar process happens when a CoQ deficiency occurs. It takes days and weeks for CoQ to rebuild its supplies from the blood, through the tissues, and then maintain sufficient supplies at a cellular level once it has been severely depleted. This process would take longer through increasing appropriate CoQ-rich nutrition than it would through adding pure CoQ supplements to the diet. CoQ's beneficial effects have to reach the very roots of the deficiency problem and work from the inside outward. Although blood levels will show an immediate boost of CoQ, the rebuilding program at the tissue, cellular, and molecular levels is gradual—billions of cells are involved throughout the body.

The action of CoQ is similar to vitamins: if the body is given more of the coenzyme than it needs it will not give your physical condition and bioenergetic potential a corresponding super-boost. *The only time that supplementation of CoQ is effective is when a deficiency state has already occurred.*

An important point to repeat is that CoQ is essential to life. Dr. Karl Folkers states that morbidity is associated with a deficiency of CoQ once it reaches a 75 percent decline, and death will definitely occur "some time" after CoQ dips under a quarter of its normal availability and heads toward zero. Research by some Japanese scientists states emphatically that death *will* occur at a 75 percent deficiency. Dr. Folkers also estimates that somewhere between a 25 and 75 percent deficiency, overt disease states will become apparent.

Deficiencies in the Heart

One of the prime essentials of a healthy heart is the ability of its muscle fibers to contract. Muscle fibers are rubber bands in reverse. A rubber band can be stretched and then it will snap back into place; you can't get a rubber band to contract and then return back to its normal length. However, the reverse is the case with muscle fibers, they can only contract and then relax back to their normal length; they will not stretch and then snap back like rubber bands.

It's for this reason that muscles always work together in pairs. To move a limb, one muscle will contract while the other relaxes, and to move it back into its original position, the reverse happens. To keep a limb in a desired position, the muscles will exert equal pressures against each other to balance the force and keep the limb stationary.

Muscles can also overlay each other like the belts on a car tire, pulling in different directions to give added strength to the overall structure. The heart is built in a similar way with sheets of muscles working against each other in sequence to create a pumping action.

But, just like the rubber band, the heart muscle fibers can lose their contractility. When this happens with the heart, its pumping function declines to the point when it can no longer sustain life. This form of myocardial failure is quite common, but the mechanism of how the impaired contractility occurs is poorly understood.

The energy factor seems to be the most obvious reason. If

the fuel source that supplies the energy to contract the muscle is reduced, then the heart's overall ability to pump will decline. One extremely important fact that cannot be ignored is that CoQ is critical to the production of cellular energy—and all muscles are made up of cells. When the availability of CoQ is reduced, cellular energy levels would be expected to fall.

In 1982 at the University Hospital in Copenhagen, Denmark, tests on patients with varying degrees of myocardial failure showed convincing results to support the conclusion that heart function deterioration is directly related to the availability of CoQ in the tissues.

Twenty-nine patients were involved in the study. Five were females, the rest males, and the average age was 43-years-old. The aim of the study was to discover if CoQ deficiencies did exist in patients with untreatable myocardial disease, and whether it would be beneficial to administer oral CoQ.

All the patients were assessed as to the severity of their problem and they were graded with numbers from the widely accepted New York Health Association (NYHA) standard for heart disease. Class I is regarded as the mildest, with class IV being the most severe.

The subjects also underwent endomyocardial biopsies to obtain samples of their heart tissue for analysis. This procedure involves inserting a probe through the main artery in the groin and working it up into the heart to "clip" a tiny sample of tissue from the left ventricle.

Results clearly showed that myocardial levels of CoQ were significantly lower in the tissue from the most severe cases, classes III and IV, when compared to the milder cases, classes I and II. The CoQ levels in the tissues of the severest cases were measured as 0.28—or nearly half what could be expected in normal, or near normal, cardiac tissue.

The study leader, Dr. Svend A. Mortensen, commented, "This study has demonstrated that myocardial tissue from patients with cardiomyopathy was significantly deficient in CoQ_{10}, especially in the advanced stages of heart failure, and showed about half the level of that found in the 'normal' myocardium."

A similar study, published in 1984, conducted by the Department of Cardiology at the Kokura Memorial Hospital, in Kitakyushu, Japan, also found remarkable deficiencies of CoQ in diseased human hearts. But this study also looked at what happened when cardiac patients were given supplements of CoQ to their normal diets. Seventy-two patients suffering from varying stages of heart disease were split into two groups. The first 36 patients, with an average age of 55 years, received 90 mg of CoQ_{10} a day for more than two weeks. The second, control, group with an average age of 53 years, was given no CoQ. Again the results showed not only a significant lack of CoQ in the diseased heart tissues, but when oral CoQ was administered the heart levels of the coenzyme in the heart increased. In the control group no beneficial effects were observed.

"It was clearly demonstrated not only that oral administration of 90 mg of CoQ_{10} could increase the serum content level, but also that of the myocardial level of patients given CoQ_{10}, was significantly higher than in control subjects," revealed research leader Dr. Masakiyo Nobuyoshi. He added, "The myocardial CoQ_{10} of patients with severe valvular disease and congestive heart failure is lower than in normal patients, and its restoration to normal concentration by oral administration might have important clinical implications in the management of these patients."

In a recent paper published in the *Proceedings of the National Academy of Sciences*, Dr. Karl Folkers together with CoQ researchers Dr. Surasi Vadhanavikit and Dr. Svend Mortensen, gave definitive proof that diseased hearts have severe CoQ deficiencies. And the researchers went one step further by suggesting that heart disease can be a direct result of CoQ deficiency.

They pointed out that extensive data since 1970, including biopsy samples from one hundred cardiac surgery patients and blood samples from one thousand cardiac patients had revealed clear deficiencies of CoQ. More than 40 patients were involved in the study, all suffering from various degrees of cardiomyopathy, varying from class I on the New York Heart Association scale of severity, to the most severe class IV. Blood samples taken from these patients showed significant deficiencies of CoQ, but, more importantly, heart tissue biopsies revealed severe deficiencies of CoQ, and the more severe the heart disease, the higher the CoQ deficiency.

For example, 6 patients in class I displayed less CoQ deficiency than the 18 patients in class II who in turn showed hearts less deficient in CoQ than the 11 class III patients. The most severe deficiencies were observed in the 8 class IV patients. CoQ was administered to the patients, who then began to display elevated blood levels of the nutrient. For ethical reasons involving taking heart tissue samples from patients responding to treatment, biopsy samples were only obtained from a sample of five patients after treatment with CoQ. The increased CoQ levels in heart tissue ranged from 20 percent to a dramatic 85 percent higher than before treatment. The following table shows these results.

TABLE I

Level of CoQ in Blood and Biopsy Samples of 5 Patients after Treatment with CoQ_{10}

Class	Blood CoQ_{10}		% increase	Myocardial CoQ		% increase
	Before	After		Before	After	
III	0.64	1.92(4.5 mo)	200	0.29	0.48	66
III	0.73	1.47(8 mo)	101	0.30	0.36	20
III	0.40	0.73(8 mo)	82	0.21	0.39	86
IV	0.95	2.59(3.5 mo)	173	0.26	0.31	19
IV	0.57	0.80(2 mo)	40	0.27	0.36	33

Dr. Folkers states, "Therapy with CoQ_{10} can result in increasing and even normalizing the myocardial levels of CoQ_{10} under optimal conditions of dosage and compliance. Therapy with CoQ_{10} can result in a profound increase both in cardiac function and in the quality of life of a failing cardiac patient. Cardiomyopathy can be substantially, but not solely, a consequence of a deficiency of CoQ_{10}."

These studies are among many which confirm the deficiency of essential CoQ in the hearts of cardiac victims. The important conclusion is that by taking oral CoQ as a daily dietary supplement, the levels of this necessary key to bioenergetics could be increased in the failing heart.

But would boosting CoQ save or prolong the lives of heart victims?

Saving Lives with CoQ

A study involving congestive heart failure appears to support the important conclusion that mild stages of the disease exhibit smaller deficiencies of CoQ than later, more severe stages, and that to be beneficial, dosages of CoQ may have to be directly proportional to the severity of the disease.

The study took place at Kitasato University School of Medicine, in Kanagawa, Japan, and was reported in 1980. Twenty cardiac patients were administered a low dose of only 30 mg a day of CoQ as a dietary supplement. The breakdown of the severity of the disease among the patients was: 3 with stage I, 12 with stage II, 4 with stage III, and one with stage IV.

At the end of the two-month study the researchers were able to report that 50 percent of the subjects exhibited noticeable improvement in their breathing ability with little or no shortness of breath; 50 percent showed enough of an improvement to be reclassified in the NYHA graded severity of the disease; more than 30 percent displayed a "remarkable" decrease in congestion revealed by chest X rays; and 30 percent displayed reduced liver enlargement.

Researcher Dr. Teruo Tsuyuasaki concluded, "In normal heart there is plenty of Coenzyme Q_{10} but in pathological states or in heart disease, there is a deficiency of Coenzyme Q_{10}. . . . It is looked upon as one of the important substances maintaining the normal cardiac function. Accordingly there is a possibility that the deficiency of Coenzyme Q_{10} may give rise to cardiac dysfunction or heart failure.

"From these results it is suggested that, in 55% of patients with congestive heart failure, clinical symptoms showed a tendency to ameliorate with the use of Coenzyme Q_{10}. However, these effects appeared frequently in patients in I or II of the NYHA classification, and such effects were hardly seen in patients in stage III or IV."

It can also be interpreted from the results of this study that 30 mg of CoQ was not a sufficiently high enough level to be of benefit to the stage III and IV patients.

But the study that follows clearly shows the superior beneficial effects of 100 mg a day in the more advanced stages of heart failure—the same stages where one would expect to find a greater deficiency of CoQ.

In Copenhagen Dr. Mortensen and his team followed up their earlier studies by selecting a small group of patients with advanced heart disease for CoQ therapy. Ten males were involved in the study, which was published in 1984. All of the patients were suffering from the severest problems and were classified as either III or IV on the NYHA scale. They were given 100 mg of oral CoQ a day. Preliminary result from the experiments showed that seven of the ten patients responded favorably to the CoQ treatment.

Again we see this remarkable correlation of around 70 to 75 percent, or three-quarters, of heart victims being helped by CoQ. It's worth recalling that Dr. Folkers's initial studies found CoQ deficiencies in 75 percent of human heart disease tissue. Obviously CoQ cannot help all cardiac victims, and it appears that a quarter of potentially fatal heart problems stem from causes other than a deficiency of CoQ.

Dr. Mortensen reported that out of the seven patients who were followed for 3 months on CoQ, five showed obvious improvement, four of them enough to reclassify them in a beneficial direction on the NYHA scale. The crucial significance of this therapy was that it appeared to "reverse" a disease state that is expected only to deteriorate.

One patient, a class IV victim, showed "remarkable" improvement beyond all expectations for a victim in such advanced cardiac disease distress. His turnaround happened just 3 weeks into the CoQ program. His blood levels of CoQ jumped from .95 at the start to 2.17 after the first month and then to 2.73 by the end of the second month on the coenzyme. The first sign of CoQ's benefit was that his difficulty in breathing, even at rest, began to diminish, and then the labored breathing disappeared altogether. He became more active and was able to undergo mild physical exercise with much less fatigue than before the CoQ therapy. The patient was reclassified a full 2 stages from a IV to a II on the severity scale. Dr. Mortensen described the therapeutic effects as "dramatic."

The Danish researcher added, "The pilot study of CoQ treatment in the severe cases of cardiomyopathy points to a deficiency state of CoQ in the myocardium in some patients and apparent effectiveness of this substance to treat myocardial disease by improving bioenergetics and increasing contractility [in heart muscle fibers]."

But can CoQ be shown to save the lives of victims of severe cardiac disease?

In the department of medical research at the Methodist

Hospital of Indiana, "no hope" class IV congestive heart failure patients were treated with CoQ as an adjunct to the traditional heart medication drug digitalis, and diuretics. The prognosis for most of the patients' ability to survive on drug therapy alone was measured in just days and weeks.

Yet another significant CoQ result was observed. An unexpected 71 percent of these "no hope" class IV victims survived for at least a year, and 62 percent were still alive 2 years after beginning the coenzyme therapy.

The comments of chief researcher Dr. W. V. Judy are worth recording: "After 180 days none of the surviving patients demonstrated positional congestive heart failure. Physical activity, if any, was limited before CoQ treatment. Many of the patients had to be physically helped to the testing table in the control studies. After 9 to 12 weeks of CoQ_{10} treatment all the responding patients were ambulatory [walking around] with significantly improved physical ability. All were able to care for themselves, indicating an improvement in the quality of life. No clinical side effects were noted with CoQ_{10} treatment."

These Indiana studies demonstrated that 80 percent of the patients had improved cardiac function after CoQ therapy—an unusually high success rate considering that the majority of these patients were already dangerously ill.

Studies of experimental drugs follow certain protocols. A double-blind crossover study is accepted as one of the strictest tests for the efficacy of a new drug. The protocol for experiments of this type usually means that the entire group of subjects are split in two, with one half receiving the test substance while the other half is administered a placebo. After a specified period the groups are swapped so that the first patients who did not receive the test drug now do, and the group that took the medicinal begin to receive placebos. What makes it "blind" is that the researchers are not aware at any stage whether the subjects are receiving the drug or the placebo. The following double-blind study illustrates the potential of CoQ to not just save lives, but to prolong the quality as well.

Dr. P. H. Langsjoen and colleagues at Scott and White Clinic, Texas A&M University in Temple, Texas, conducted such an experiment with 19 patients, all in the most severe III and IV classes of primary heart failure. Another indication of the seriousness of the conditions of these patients was the fact that 25 were originally selected but one died at the beginning of the study and another was accepted for a heart transplant during its course. Four other patients were excluded for various technical and ethical reasons.

The subjects comprised 11 males and 8 females, with an average age of 63 years, who had all previously had at least one heart attack. They were divided into two groups, one of 8 patients and the other 11. Their CoQ deficiencies were measured by the levels of the nutrient in their blood. The first group received 33 mg of CoQ three times a day, while the rest were given placebos. After 12 weeks the situations were reversed.

The results were highly encouraging and showed in yet another clinical study that the levels of CoQ can be significantly boosted by taking oral CoQ supplements. Put another way, CoQ can act as a treatment for serious heart disease.

In each of the first eight subjects to take CoQ, blood levels of the coenzyme were increased after the administration of CoQ, and declined once they were switched to placebos. In the second group of 11, only one person failed to show a blood level increase in CoQ once the group changed over from the placebos.

Dr. Langsjoen reported, "These patients, steadily worsening and expected to die within 2 years under conventional therapy, generally showed an extraordinary clinical improvement, indicating that CoQ_{10} therapy might extend the lives of such patients. Eighteen of 19 patients reported clinical improvement after the treatment period, manifested almost entirely by increased general activity tolerance in parallel with improvement in cardiac function."

In the carefully measured words of a research scientist, Dr. Langsjoen states that a CoQ deficiency is "likely a factor in the functional abnormality" of severe heart disease, and is "just possibly" instrumental in the root cause of chronic myocardial disease.

But Langsjoen was categorical in his summary of the test results and the lack of any side effects associated with CoQ therapy. "Oral CoQ_{10} is a safe and effective therapy for chronic myocardial disease. We believe that the remarkable clinical improvement of cardiomyopathy patients during CoQ_{10} treatment results from improved bioenergetics which supports improved cardiac function."

Impedance Cardiography

Impedance cardiography is absolutely noninvasive technology—a revolutionary new method to assess heart function. It's no longer necessary to make incisions, insert probes or wires into the heart, squirt dyes into the bloodstream, or resort to any of the other techniques previously associated with successfully obtaining an accurate picture of the heart's health, or lack of it.

The technique—its scientific name is transthoracic electrical impedance—is relatively new and has been developed over the past two decades to replace many of the less inviting and less accurate methods of heart function measurement. The system gauges cardiac output and stroke volume, two of the most significant mechanical functions of the heart. Cardiac output is the total volume of blood being pumped from the heart and is measured in liters per minute. Stroke volume is the amount of blood pumped in one heartbeat, and this is read in milliliters per beat. From these calculations we can determine the contractility of the heart, which is called the Heather Index.

Dr. Folkers and his team of heart scientists sampled individuals aged between 19 and 34 years and came up with the following averages for the healthy heart: cardiac output, 7.28 liters/minute; stroke volume 105 milliliters/heartbeat; and 13 for the Heather Index. These figures are well worth remembering when comparing the impedance cardiography readings of diseased hearts and the results after treatment with CoQ.

At first glance impedance cardiography may appear frightening, but it is simple, painless, harmless, and noninvasive. A circular electrode, which generates about 40 KHz of alternating current, is applied around the entire forehead. A second aluminum adhesive band is placed around the upper abdomen. Two additional inner electrode bands are positioned around the neck and the thorax.

In addition, body weight, height, and the distance between the electrodes are all taken into account. The simple "magic" of the technique is that it accurately measures the heart's function by analyzing tiny variations in electrical voltage between the electrode sensors, which are then fed into a computer which calculates the differentials into readings for the cardiac output, stroke volume, and Heather Index.

With traditional invasive methods of assessing the heart's performance a patient would have to be hospitalized. Because of the need to enter the body there were actual surgical techniques that were time-consuming and often painful. This alone meant severe limitations on how often measurements could be taken.

Impedance cardiography can be conducted on an out-patient basis over a period of 30 minutes and, day by day, this can amount to hundreds of individual measurements of the heart and to analyzing thousands of single heartbeats.

Table II shows typical readouts for a control group of healthy individuals as measured by impedance cardiography. Table III shows the measurements taken for a group of cardiac patients at the start and during CoQ treatment. Both sets of data are from Dr. Folkers research group at the Institute for Biomedical Research at the University of Texas, in Austin.

TABLE II

Cardiac Data on a Control Group by Impedance Cardiography

Age	Sex	Cardiac Output	Stroke Volume	Heather Index
23	F	6.05	95.60	10.06
29	F	5.75	88.25	18.40
30	M	6.34	97.65	13.80
33	M	6.98	89.60	17.00
20	M	7.59	124.50	13.70
34	M	6.74	88.85	10.15
19	M	9.43	121.50	14.05
29	M	8.44	111.50	16.50
25	M	8.24	129.00	11.35
Mean*		7.28	105.16	13.89

*When making comparisons with the next chart, you may want to refer back to these mean scores, being the averages for healthy individuals.

By comparing the charts of the healthy group, it is obvious that the cardiac patients' heart performance values are much lower. When CoQ treatment was introduced to the group in the second table, it clearly shows that in almost every reading there was a distinct improvement.

TABLE III

Data from Treatment of Cardiac Patients with CoQ
Daily dosages of CoQ were 60–100 mg.

Age	Sex	Period (months)	Cardiac Output		Stroke Volume		Heather Index	
			1st*	2nd*	1st*	2nd*	1st*	2nd*
75	M	9	3.59	4.83	45.00	59.65	10.10	10.56
66	M	4	2.42	3.23	24.70	43.53	7.70	9.24
51	M	8	2.43	3.64	26.40	38.82	4.70	5.80
58	M	6	3.06	3.65	43.55	55.05	6.68	5.87
59	F	5	2.57	3.03	28.80	36.37	12.90	12.32
71	M	5	2.05	2.89	20.95	32.05	4.99	7.76
38	M	6	3.65	3.25	45.30	51.80	7.30	7.39
78	M	6	1.99	2.56	28.20	30.65	6.18	6.45

*1st means before initiation of treatment and 2nd was a measurement taken during treatment.

Individual Case Histories

The obvious value of impedance cardiography becomes apparent in CoQ research when its realized that hundreds of different readings of heart data can be made on a daily basis for a single individual.

This is of critical importance because it can accurately show the ongoing beneficial effects after a regimen of CoQ treatment has been started. And it allows the results to be given not only on an overall group basis, but to narrow the findings down to individual patients, with a comprehensive view of the heart that was previously unheard of. These instant pictures of heart function reveal CoQ's benefits in a very personalized way.

A joint research project, published in 1984, between the Hospital of Rehabilitation in Bornheim-Merten and the University of Bonn, both in West Germany, provided a unique look into the diseased heart and the benefits of CoQ. Twenty-four patients suffering from congestive heart failure were involved in a double-blind crossover study. Twelve received three doses of 33 mg of CoQ per day, and the other half of the group were given placebos. Then the situations were reversed.

Here are some of the individual results (the study is ongoing and the final results are not available as of this writing):

Patient R.J., a 66-year-old female, entered the study and was randomly selected for the placebo group. Immediately prior to participating her cardiac output varied between 2.7 and 2.9. The stroke volume readings showed from a high of 45 to a low of 38.

At the start of the study her cardiac parameters showed a very slight beneficial increase (possibly due to hospital care), but after 9 weeks on placebos her cardiac output measured 2.3 and stroke volume around 34. Her condition was, if anything, clearly deteriorating.

Patient M.G., a 73-year-old female, had rapidly declining cardiac output and stroke volume. Immediately prior to the start of the study her cardiac output had fallen from an average of 3.5 to less than 2.5. Her stroke volume had plummeted from around 40 to just over 20. In the hospital environment with good nutrition, care, and lack of stress, her condition stabilized, and for the next 15 weeks she took placebos with the result being minor improvement with cardiac output levels returning to an average of 3 and stroke volume to around 35.

After week 15 she was crossed over to receive CoQ. Her heart parameters began to improve dramatically. By week 20 her cardiac output had jumped to 4.5 and her stroke volume to almost 50.

Patient W. S., a 73-year-old male, entered the program and received 100 mg of CoQ from day 1. Immediately prior to starting CoQ therapy his cardiac output had dropped slightly from 3.25 to 3. His stroke volume had dipped from 40 to just over 30.

By the 10th week on CoQ his cardiac output had consistently risen to hit 6, while his stroke volume shot up to almost 90. At this point the patient's daily dosage of CoQ was reduced to 33 mg. Within 7 weeks his cardiac output dropped to 4.5 and the stroke volume to almost 70.

The patient was then returned to full CoQ therapy of 100 mg, and within two weeks his cardiac output and stroke volume had bounced back to the highs achieved before CoQ had been reduced.

The previous two case histories could be considered as dramatic proof of the beneficial effect of CoQ as a treatment for the diseased and failing heart. The next case we include is considered by the German researchers as more typical of the average response during CoQ therapy.

Patient C.D., a 73-year-old female, entered the study with cardiac output readings of approximately 3.4, and her stroke volume was around 60. She received CoQ for the next 15 weeks.

By week 6 her cardiac output measurement peaked at 6 and her stroke volume at almost 100. Her condition then began to stabilize with a small decrease in the heart function values. By the end of the 13th week her cardiac output remained steady at 4.5 and her stroke volume at just under 80.

When analyzing patient C.D. as experiencing a typical beneficial effect from CoQ, it is important to note that her heart values increased and peaked early on in therapy, and then lowered and remained at a constant plateau, which was still greatly improved over initial cardiac output and stroke volume findings.

In the more severe cases where the disease had progressed further, it could be argued that the CoQ deficiency was greater and therefore, once CoQ was introduced, the beneficial result would be more dramatic giving an enhanced picture of CoQ's effectiveness; the more profound the need, the more obvious the end result.

The study group's leader, Dr. W. Schneeberger, commented, "What can be seen at the moment with patients undergoing CoQ_{10} treatment is the increase in their well-being. They all show an improvement in their general condition, an increase in physical capacity, less dyspnea [difficulty in breathing], less nocturia [incontinence of urine at night], and less oedema [swelling of tissues]. All patients observed under CoQ_{10} treatment show a statistically significant increase in cardiac output and stroke volume. In general a greater physical and mental fitness can be observed in these patients."

In the United States, impedance cardiography is widely gaining acceptance among cardiologists, and Dr. Karl Folkers has recently released data on cardiac patients who received CoQ while being monitored by the new heart measuring technique. Seven of the eight heart patients in his study displayed significant increases in their cardiac output ability, reveals Dr. Folkers.

The data on a typical patient reads: "Patient G.A. was 75-years-old. Measurements of his cardiac parameters on six separate days gave a mean value of cardiac output which was 3.59 and a mean stroke volume of 45. On treatment, his cardiac output became 4.83 and his stroke volume became 59."

Dr. Folkers adds, "If a patient has a myocardial deficiency of CoQ_{10}, and the deficiency is corrected by oral CoQ_{10} so the heart pumps more effectively, it is not likely that more effective pumping will be maintained when oral CoQ_{10} is terminated, because the dietary and metabolic conditions giving rise to the deficiency of CoQ_{10} will still be present. Consequently, therapy with CoQ_{10} for cardiac patients may be for prolonged periods and even for a lifetime."

Latest Studies

If the proposal for long-term therapy is combined with "no hope" cardiac cases and the results are still looking good months later, it should prove beyond doubt the efficacy of CoQ treatments.

In Copenhagen, Dr. Mortensen, with guidance from Folkers's research group from Austin, has now shown—and this was reported in late 1985—that long term improvements can be maintained, even with major myocardial failure which is impervious to the best of traditional therapy and drugs.

Twelve patients were involved in this landmark research at the Municipal Hospital in Aarhus, Denmark. All were suffering advanced heart failure, and all were given 100 mg of CoQ daily as an oral supplement to their regular diets. Emphasizes Dr. Mortensen, "They were all showing insufficient response to classical therapy with diuretics and digitalis."

The first confirmations of CoQ's effectiveness came within an average of 30 days, during which time 8 of the 12 (67%) showed definite clinical improvement. "Subjectively, the patients felt less tired, their general activity tolerance increased and dyspnoea [difficulty breathing] at rest disappeared," reports Dr. Mortensen. "There were obvious signs of decreased right-sided hepatic congestion. The heart rate fell significantly, and the heart volume decreased in the eight responders. A significant reduction in the left atrial size was registered, suggesting a reduced preload of the left ventricle."

Furthermore, constant heart performance monitoring showed greatly increased myocardial performance.

To leave no doubt that CoQ was responsible, and only the administration of CoQ, the researchers began to withdraw selected patients off CoQ therapy. The results were dramatic. Patients heart conditions immediately began to deteriorate. They were returned immediately to CoQ therapy. Confirms Dr. Mortensen, "Preliminary CoQ_{10} withdrawal results showed severe clinical relapse with subsequent improvement on CoQ_{10} reinstatement, supporting the interpretation that treatment of these patients corrected a myocardial deficiency of CoQ_{10} and increased contractility [of the heart muscle]. Hence CoQ_{10} appears to be an effective therapeutic agent in advanced cases of heart failure. This is an attractive circumvention of the traditional principles of therapy: supporting the myocardium directly by ameliorating a supposed underlying mitochondrial dysfunction [exhausted bioenergetics]."

At the writing of their report, the Danish and American researchers had followed the progress of the patients for a full seven months, with not only dramatic improvements, but also without the loss of one life.

Another very recent study yet again confirmed the effectiveness of CoQ in treating patients with chronic myocardial disease—all with either NYHA classes III or IV severity of disease levels.

At Scott & White Memorial Hospital, in Temple, Texas, 18 out of 19 cardiac patients in a double-blind crossover study displayed remarkable benefits once introduced to 100 mg of oral CoQ each day. Research leader Dr. P. H. Langsjoen revealed in a 1985 report, "All had either low or borderline levels of CoQ_{10} in their blood, and showed a significant change into the normal range with oral CoQ_{10} replacement. Eighteen patients reported improvement in activity tolerance with therapy. Combined clinical observations, stroke volume measured by impedance cardiography, and ejection fractions calculated from systolic time intervals, all showed significant improvement in parallel with CoQ_{10} administration." Dr. Langsjoen added enthusiastically, "This application of the principles of bioenergetics introduces a promising new dimension to the study and treatment of the complex problems of myocardial failure."

An Encouraging Future

There is little doubt from the results of studies utilizing CoQ as a treatment for advanced heart failure, that it works. The addition of simple CoQ supplements to the diet have been shown to improve the pumping capacity of the ailing heart, and therefore prolong lives that may well have been lost within days or weeks if CoQ had not been administered.

But prolonging existence may not be desirable if there is no quality to that life. With CoQ one of the most obvious factors is the great improvement of not only the physical but also the mental well-being of heart patients, whether they are elderly or in middle age.

Patients who were hardly able to move because of congestive heart failure and the extreme distress it brings to breathing, even while at rest, have been able to walk again after CoQ treatments. Patients whose conditions were so severe that they even needed assistance to get onto an examination table are able once more to look to a new, active future through CoQ.

After the introduction of oral CoQ to their diets, patients have been able to easily outlive previous life expectations; cardiac functions improved, and for many they were again able to move, talk, laugh, and perform physical activities they never thought would be possible again. And most important, they had a new will to live and were able to care for themselves once more.

These previous studies have concentrated on the most dire forms of heart disease, on treatment, and on prolonging life with Coenzyme Q_{10}. But this encouraging story doesn't stop here.

In the vast realm of heart problems there are not just the potentially terminal cases, but also those with less severe heart damage, which can be equally distressing: angina pectoris for one, arteriosclerosis for another, and the failure of not the heart itself, but the other systems connected to it and its internal components, such as valves. Can these also be helped by CoQ?

The answer is undoubtedly yes. CoQ studies now reveal that not only can this essential nutrient be utilized to treat the heart, but also to protect it from further damage, aid and improve the effects of heart surgery, protect the heart against potentially toxic drugs, improve its function, and even shield it prophylactically.

CHAPTER 6

•

Protecting the Heart

Some readers of this book have had heart attacks and they don't even know it! Most people tend to imagine a heart attack as a sudden excruciating pain in the chest that completely incapacitates the victim and causes immediate death. This can happen, but the majority of heart attacks display a longer process.

Heart attacks have many clinical faces. In fact, no two heart attacks may be exactly identical because of the varying degrees of damage that they can inflict on the cardiac organ. While the symptoms of an attack can also differ, the end product, the survivability factor, is measured by exactly how much tissue and how many cells in the heart muscle have died. A massive coronary that proves fatal, has caused death because inevitably not enough healthy heart tissue has survived to be capable of continuing the pumping process.

No heart attack can be considered minor, but people can suffer an attack, even numerous ones, and not realize they have experienced a coronary. The fleeting intense pain in the chest is often of such short duration that the victim might pass it off as indigestion, a muscle spasm, or even an attack of gas. The damage that has occurred to the heart is so small that it will display no significant symptoms or aftereffects. The person will most probably continue their life-style without knowing their heart has issued a deadly warning.

This type of unrecognized attack is no phantom. Although no apparent disability will be present after the event, it may be detected later, even years later, by a trained medical professional through standard physiological tests in the doctor's office. Its legacy will be a small portion of useless, deceased heart muscle.

A question this type of attack raises is: At what point do we consider administration of CoQ as protection for the heart, and when do we view it as treatment?

Because of an increasing public awareness of heart attack symptoms, and the importance of post-attack life-style changes, an increasing number of cardiac victims are surviving today. This means that there are more opportunities to consider not only treating a present condition but protecting against a further occurrence.

When CoQ is utilized as a therapeutic agent after a heart disorder has been diagnosed, its functional role is as both a protector and a treatment; it is being used as treatment to correct a deficiency, and prophylactically to ward off the possibility of the deficiency recurring.

The Attack

There are numerous factors that may contribute to the potentially lethal condition we term a heart attack, among them are congenital heart defects, rheumatic heart disease, atherosclerosis, and high blood pressure. We will deal with these individually, but for the moment let's consider the mechanism of the attack itself.

Like all muscles the heart is totally dependent on an abundant supply of blood. This is its lifeline and is supplied by the coronary arteries that run through the heart muscle itself. Paradoxically it is the heart's own job to supply its own blood, in a self-sustaining circulation.

But coronary arteries can become old and fragile, and even collapse. More often they become narrowed through build-ups of fatty deposits known as plaque on the inside walls of the vessels. When an artery becomes totally blocked, its ability to supply the heart muscle with fresh oxygenated blood is lost, and consequently the portion of the heart muscle being fed oxygen, and other nutrients, by this vessel begins to die.

In severely narrowed vessels the chances that blood clots can form and block the flow of blood are great. This is referred to as a coronary thrombosis, coronary occlusion, or myocardial infarction.

An infarction is the death of a section of tissue because the blood supply has been cut off. The myocardium is the muscular middle layer of the heart. A myocardial infarction is, therefore, the death of that portion of tissue in the heart. A thrombosis occurs when a vessel is blocked, or occluded, by a clot, which also cuts off blood supply and can lead to an infarct. Ischemia means a deficiency of the blood supply. Hypoxia is a lack of oxygen to tissues, which can be a direct result of ischemia.

The warning signals of a full-fledged heart attack are listed by the American Heart Association as follows:

• Uncomfortable pressure, fullness, squeezing, or pain in the center of the chest, lasting two minutes or longer.
• Spreading of pain to shoulders, neck, or arms.
• Severe pain, dizziness, fainting, sweating, nausea, or short-ness of breath may also occur.

Not all these signals are always present together in a heart attack. If you are unsure, don't wait, don't take chances, get help immediately.

How the Heart Can Save Itself

The heart does have its own fail-safe method of protecting itself when a heart attack occurs. It is known as collateral circulation—the heart's own compensatory plan in which minor blood vessels begin to supply blood to the area of the heart served by the blocked artery. These small collateral vessels open up to detour more blood to the damaged area of the heart. In some cases this protective process may start to happen as the major artery begins to narrow and before it is fully blocked.

If the amount of the heart threatened by the shutdown is not too large, the compensatory effect of the collateral circu-lation can prevent serious injury and ischemic death of the muscle tissues. But clearly this will also put an overload on a presumably not too healthy cardiac system and also a drain on its bioenergetic capabilities.

Consider the point that if the heart is already suffering from a serious deficiency of its bioenergetic capabilities, even with the saving graces of collateral circulation compensation it may still be in jeopardy.

It now becomes apparent that if we can improve the de-pleted bioenergetics with the aid of additional CoQ supple-ments to the tissue and cells, we can help strengthen the failing heart by increasing its energy efficiency. If the lack of intrinsic bioenergy was indeed a result of a CoQ deficiency, then we are not only strengthening the heart, but also protecting against the possibility of the heart not being able to cope with another attack, which might prove to be fatal the next time.

From Mouse to Man

There's a world of difference between mice and men, but essentially the minuscule physical processes of mice are very much like our own, they're just laid out differently and on a smaller scale. So, what happens at the cellular level in an organ of a mouse can very well reflect what we might expect to happen in a human organ cell.

Animals differ from humans in the foods they eat, the nutrients they require, and the amounts that they consume. But animals' hearts and human hearts have one thing in common, they need CoQ to survive.

So, animal models, including rats, rabbits, and dogs, in the controlled laboratory surrounding can give a good indication of how we might expect CoQ to act on the human body. It's not exact, and allowances have to be made for size variations and other factors not in common, but on the whole, animals as tiny as mice can provide valuable information that we can then interpret for the human condition.

We would never perform a biopsy on a healthy human heart and test it in the laboratory. With animals specially bred for the purpose of medical experimentation, we do have this valuable option of being able to take even a beating, living organ and examine it right down to the finest detail.

At the Tsukuba Research Laboratories and the Department of Medicine at the National Defense Medical College, in Japan, research scientists decided to attempt to determine the effect of CoQ on hypoxic cellular damage in cardiac muscle, which simply means the damage caused by the lack of oxygen to heart tissue, as in a heart attack.

Heart cells are such that even when they are isolated individually they still beat out the rhythm of a healthy heart. Heart cells from mice embryos were selected. Scientists in Japan had managed to develop a process whereby ischemic myocardial injury could be duplicated in individual animal heart cells and this could act as a model for what would be expected to happen in the human heart.

The mouse heart cells were kept in unique life-sustaining solutions where they were able to continue a healthy beat as if they were still in the heart. After some 48 hours, allowing the cells to acclimatize to their new situation, the oxygen supply to these cells was gradually decreased and consequently cellular respiration (part of the bioenergetic process) was inhibited. This experimental process successfully mimics the effects of a heart attack when oxygen is deprived from cardiac muscle and its cells.

This fascinating research took a two-pronged approach and compared the actions of CoQ to the actions of a drug, a known cardiac stimulator. The first phase of the experiment might be likened to the treatment of a heart attack in progress. The next phase was to look at any beneficial effects CoQ may have had in protecting the heart cells from further damage during the period in which they were deprived of life-sustaining oxygen.

While the cells were undergoing the effects of hypoxia (lack of oxygen), and could be considered to be dying, they received the drug and, later, the CoQ. What the scientists saw under the microscope was rather remarkable.

When the drug was administered, the beats of the cells dipped to approximately 83 beats per minute for 5 minutes and then increased and leveled out at 102 beats for the next 60 minutes. CoQ was then introduced in three increasing concentrations—100, 200, and 400 ug/ml, respectively (if the size and terminology of the dosage seems confusing—it actually means micrograms per millileter—the important factor to remember is the numerical figures). The increase in the beats corresponding to the dosage was impressive: they jumped to 129, 144, and 161 in direct relation to the increasing amounts of CoQ administered.

The nutrient was clearly having a profound effect on the ability of single heart cells to increase their beating ability to, presumably, better utilize what little oxygen was available to them. What the researchers also found was that before they starved the cells of oxygen they could expect to see an average of 2 irregular beats per minute (a natural effect under the experimental conditions). As the hypoxia took effect, the irregular beats increased to 5 after 30 minutes, and 7 after an hour. The effects of the lack of oxygen was obviously taking its toll and heading toward an increase of irregular beats that would no longer perform the rhythmic pumping action of the heart, and ultimately could be expected to be unable to sustain life.

But after CoQ was added the irregular beats dramatically decreased and returned to the expected norm of about 2 per minute. The researchers concluded that in a heart attack scenario, CoQ not only increases the function of the heart cell, but also protects it from further damage from lack of oxygen.

Two theories were offered by the researchers as possibilities for CoQ's protective role. The first was that it acted directly at the mitochondria level by changing the bioenergetic respiratory chain of events, by either conserving energy or reducing the need for it, and thus preventing tissue death. The second proposal was that CoQ may act on the membrane of individual heart cells, "sealing them off" from the effects of killing toxic chemicals that would build up as a result of the hypoxia in the tissue.

Similar studies of CoQ's beneficial protective effects were performed at the Jikei University School of Medicine and the Yamanashi Medical College, in Japan. Live hearts and lungs were removed intact from rats and kept alive on an artificial respirator. The researchers were able to control the flow of blood and instigate the effects of ischemia (lack of blood flow) to the heart.

What they discovered also demonstrated the likelihood that CoQ acts protectively on the myocardial cell membrane because only hearts treated with CoQ supplements were able to survive the ischemic process without significant injury.

Another Japanese experiment compared the action of CoQ with the heart drug methylprednisolone (MP), which is known to help reduce the damaging effect of heart ischemia and aid the organ in recovering function. One marker the scientists were able to use was the fact that injured heart tissue muscle fibers release a specific factor known as LCII into the blood stream: the higher the level of the factor detected after a heart attack, the greater the damage has been to heart muscle tissues.

Researchers from Faculty of Medicine, at the University of Tokyo, took 30 experimental dogs and divided them into three groups. Using a surgical technique, a main coronary artery was closed to result in a myocardial infarction. One group of ten dogs was used as a control while a second group received CoQ supplementation before and after the artificially induced heart attack. The third group received the drug MP. Constant measurements of their blood level contents were taken.

Ten days later the dogs were sacrificed and their hearts examined for damage. There was little difference to distinguish between the sizes of the areas affected by the initial infarction. The control group showed 10.5 percent of affected tissue, the MP group 10.2 percent, and the CoQ group 9.8 percent.

But the significant surprise was that the CoQ treated dogs had displayed much reduced levels of the telltale LCII factor. The control group showed a factor of 1212 of LCII release over 10 days, the MP group 1129, and the CoQ dogs only 814—a clear sign that the CoQ stimulated hearts had weathered the attacks with far less damage to the muscle fibers of the heart.

The researchers concluded that CoQ had not only helped to slightly reduce the area affected by the attack, but prevented it from spreading further, and dramatically reduced the tissue damage that could have occurred.

Previously stated was the fact that CoQ is crucial in the production of ATP, the biological energy component, at the cellular level. An experiment performed by the Cardiopulmonary Division at the Keio University School of Medicine, in Japan, probed to see if there was among the benefits of CoQ's protection, one which preserved the valuable ATP. There was!

Reporting the experiments in 1985, *Cardiovascular Research*, a prestigious journal of the British Medical Association, revealed that when heart attacks were induced in dogs that had been pretreated with CoQ, they showed more preservation of ATP than dogs that had received no CoQ. Coenzyme Q dogs displayed 3.25 ATP in the ischemic myocardium while nontreated dogs showed 2.96.

Researchers in the Cardiothoracic Institute at the University of London, England, reported in 1980 that they had tested the ability to protect the heart against injury during an attack, but this time in rabbits. Some of the animals were given CoQ boosting supplements for 7 days before the series of experiments, which included induced heart attack, were performed. The study leader, Dr. Winifred G. Nayler, reported conclusively, "Our results show that Coenzyme Q_{10} can be used prophylactically to protect the myocardium against the deleterious effects of ischaemia."

The American Journal of Cardiovascular Pharmacology reported in 1982 on Japanese experiments that reaffirmed the capacity of CoQ to protect the heart when it is deprived of oxygen. Again the subjects were rabbits, some of which were fed intravenously with CoQ supplements for 3 days prior, while others received no CoQ. Then hypoxia was induced in the rabbit's hearts for 60 minutes and they were later analyzed to find out how the CoQ hearts had performed.

The journal's summary commented, "These results indicate that the prior and repetitive administration of CoQ_{10} may protect cardiac muscles from functional deterioration induced by hypoxia, suggesting a beneficial effect of this substance on the metabolism of the energy-depleted myocardium."

There are now literally hundreds of experiments involving animals that have proved the action of CoQ to reduce the amount of permanent cardiac injury during a heart attack and also to go on protecting the organ, which may not have previously had the beneficial prophylactic effects of CoQ due to a natural deficiency in its own tissues—a condition especially manifest in the heart.

Levels of CoQ in Human Heart Failure

Previously, human experiments had shown that the heart in distress did indeed benefit from additional oral supplements of CoQ. But it had not been conclusively established that the heart was actually absorbing the additional CoQ and where it was going. The opportunity to do this arose on a grand scale with a study at the Osaka National Hospital involving 74 heart patients who were about to undergo open heart cardiac surgery to correct valvular heart disease.

Because the patients were to undergo the radical surgery, it was an opportunity to take tissue samples from the insides of the heart, which could then be evaluated in the laboratory. They were broadly divided into two groups: one group consisted of 44 patients who were given CoQ orally in doses of 60 to 90 mg per day for 7 days prior to surgery, and the remainder acted as a control group who were not treated with CoQ.

The main conclusion to be drawn from this study was that

the more severe the heart disease, the higher the myocardial uptake of orally administered CoQ. In diseased hearts that received no CoQ, the levels of already existing CoQ were found to be significantly lower, and the reductions were in direct relationship to the severity of the heart problem.

The biopsy tissue samples taken by the cardiovascular surgeons were obtained from the right atrium, the right ventricle, and the left ventricle. And they produced an illuminating, although still not fully understood, finding—the heart's CoQ needs vary in the different pumping chambers!

Reported the researchers: The right ventricles showed average physiological levels of CoQ calculated at a figure of 107.3; the left ventricles, 79.1; and for the right atriums, 53.3.

Another interesting finding confirmed that CoQ had been absorbed in the three heart chambers of people who had been given CoQ, but a curious anomaly became apparent— the levels of additional CoQ uptake was most significant in the left ventricles only. This and other findings on the different CoQ values found in the individual heart chambers raises an important question: Why should one part of the heart need (or lack) more CoQ than another? This intriguing issue has not been answered yet.

CoQ and Drug Combinations

There's one big problem that researchers always come up against when designing a protocol to test a new untried therapy on extremely sick patients—you cannot ethically deprive them of other tried and tested drugs which may bring them relief! This causes a dilemma, no matter how much confidence there is in a drug to be tested, is it right to deprive a person of a known, possibly lifesaving, drug even though it might not be having any apparent effect? The answer is no, while there is life there's hope, and the already proven drug might be what eventually prevents the patient from crossing the line between life and death.

The answer to this vexing problem is to try to find a group of patients who are showing no response to all the available conventional treatments, and then devise a protocol to introduce your drug as an adjunct therapy.

This method was used by researchers from the Department of Internal Medicine at Kyoto University, in Japan, with heart patients at the Hyogo Kenritsu Amagasaki Hospital. Fifteen patients were studied from November 1980 to March 1981. They had various forms of heart failure and most had already had two or three prior hospital admissions for their conditions. They had also shown a lack of response to conventional treatments.

During the period of the study all these desperately ill patients were given placebos and then switched to 90 mg of CoQ therapy a day, or vice versa, so that the effects of CoQ versus no CoQ could be accurately measured.

The researchers reported exciting beneficial effects. The following are two case histories of patients that the researchers considered "representative" of the study.

Case Y.M.: The patient was a 56-year-old male. He had been hospitalized several times because of recurrent ventricular arrhythmia, heart failure, and angina pectoris, which resisted conventional treatment. Tests revealed severe disease affecting three vessels and an electrocardiogram showed a severely erratic heartbeat. After CoQ treatment his heartbeat returned to within accepted parameters, and cardiac output and stroke volume improved. Before treatment he was confined to bed most of the time, but after treatment he was capable of visiting the hospital as an outpatient.

Case F.M.: The patient was a 45-year-old male. He had typical effort angina. Two major cardiac vessels were completely blocked but he was not suffering from miocardial infarction due to the effectiveness of collateral circulation. After CoQ treatment, exercise test scores greatly improved, together with noticeable improvement in cardiac output and stroke volume.

The researchers concluded that in view of the beneficial facts associated with CoQ "the administration of CoQ_{10} at a dose level of 90 mg per day seems to provide a safe and rational adjunct to the therapy for pathological heart muscle."

Arrhythmias

When the heart starts to beat erratically we call it an arrhythmia. It's like an orchestra playing out of time, a clock unable to keep correct time because it slows down or speeds up, or the gears of an automobile transmission that slip or won't mesh properly.

On the whole, the effect is not devastating, but it contributes to overall decreased performance. And if the condition continues to worsen, and the heartbeats become increasingly erratic, the entire system can grind to a halt.

The rhythmic beats of the heart are in strict sequence and controlled by minute electrical impulses from a natural heart pacemaker. When irregularities occur it is generally because the heart's electrical pathways have been blocked or "short-circuited." Drugs can help to restore the natural rhythm, or surgeons can implant a battery operated pacemaker with wires that attach to the heart and relay impulses at the required rate.

It has long been believed by scientists, like Dr. Karl Folkers, that a disruption of the natural bioenergetics of the heart through a lack of CoQ can result in disturbances of the organ's electrical impulses. As bioenergy and the heart's electrical output may be created from the same cellular fuels, it hardly seems surprising that a deficiency of CoQ can disrupt the heart's natural pacemaking ability.

In a series of tests conducted in 1981, Dr. Folkers and co-workers from the Institute for Biomedical Research, at the University of Texas in Austin, followed the progress of a group of patients with coronary artery disease and hypertension who were being treated with CoQ.

A noticeable beneficial increase in the patient's cardiac output and stroke volume was recorded by impedance cardiography during treatment periods of 2 months or longer. But a new phenomenon was also noticed among six patients who had displayed severe arrhythmias—their irregular heartbeats were reduced or disappeared altogether.

The results using CoQ tend to speak for themselves. Out of the six patients only one showed little response to CoQ therapy. Not included in these individual reports were the many other heart parameters, including cardiac output and stroke volumes, that also showed significant benefits from CoQ.

The reader may question whether the traditional medications received by most of the six patients might have contributed to their improved arrhythmia conditions. The fact still remains that the arrhythmia victims had been on these medications for prolonged periods, and the significant changes in their arrhythmias were not noticeable until after CoQ had been introduced. In addition, two patients had received no other treatments prior to the introduction of CoQ, yet they also showed improvement.

Boosting the Performance of the Already Stricken Heart

Once the heart has undergone the trauma of attack, or the effects of serious disease states, can its remaining health not only be continued but boosted? The answer appears to be yes, according to studies conducted at the Free University in Brussels, Belgium, and published in 1984.

Dr. J. H. P. Venfraechem and colleagues had already shown that they were able to boost the cardiac performance of healthy young men by the addition of CoQ alone. Without the benefits of exercise programs improving cardiac performance, the researchers found that sedentary men could obtain the energized cardiac effects of continuous exercise programs by just taking CoQ.

With that in mind the researchers turned to heart victims to try and duplicate their results. The study involved 11 patients whose average age was 58 years. During the test period they maintained the traditional forms of drug therapy that had been prescribed for them.

The first step of the study was to test their maximum aerobic output on an electromagnetic bicycle ergometer to establish their abilities before CoQ administration. After 12 weeks of CoQ therapy, at 100 mg a day, their hearts' abilities to tolerate exercise were measured again and compared to the original tests. The results were impressive. The statistics showed an average increase of 20 percent across the board in the heart's hemodynamic ability to pump blood; its pumping capacity and energetics were without doubt greatly improved. Not only that, but the researchers recorded a 12 percent increase in the muscle power of the heart—valuable strength had also been boosted.

When considering the findings, remember that these patients are heart victims whose most vital organ had been "badly wounded." If anything, their outlook for the future could be expected to have been a continuous struggle with the heart's abilities gradually deteriorating.

To further prove the benefits of CoQ, unknown to the patients, their CoQ therapy was substituted with placebo for a further 12 weeks. The result? In every single case the newly acquired benefits gradually disappeared and dropped to the levels first recorded prior to CoQ therapy.

Relieving Painful Angina

Suffering with angina is similar to experiencing the pain of a mini heart attack without the usual, potentially fatal after-effects. The angina victim feels his pain when the heart is stressed, and this may be an act as simple as running a short distance, carrying a heavy bag of groceries, or cleaning the family car. But otherwise he can lead a normal life-style without suffering any symptoms.

The condition is, however, a serious form of heart disease and caused by constricted arteries. The debilitating chest pain is called angina pectoris, and during an angina attack it can be severe enough to completely immobilize the victim.

Most angina victims can perform little or no exercise. The still open but narrowed arteries of the heart are not able to deliver the additional oxygen that the heart muscle requires during times of emotional excitement or unusual physical exertion—even though it may be adequate to meet the heart's normal needs.

The *American Journal of Cardiology* reported in 1985 on the therapeutic benefits of CoQ in treating and increasing the quality of the lives of angina sufferers. The published study was conducted by scientists at the Department of Internal Medicine at Hamamatsu University, in Japan.

The researchers studied 12 men and 2 women whose ages ranged from 45 to 66 years, and who all suffered from chronic stable angina. A double-blind crossover procedure was used and multistage treadmill exercise tests gauged increased exercise tolerance.

Results showed that after 4 weeks of taking daily doses of 150 mg of CoQ, the patients showed an average decrease from 5.3 angina attacks to 2.5 attacks. There was also a corresponding decrease in the necessity for nitroglycerin medication that halved from a need for 2.6 tablets to 1.3 over the 4 week period. Exercise performance increased from 345 seconds with placebo to 406 seconds during CoQ treatment. Another interesting finding was that the duration before a definite ischemic process (lack of blood) could be recorded was 196 seconds with placebo, and raised to 284 with CoQ.

The researchers stated, "This study suggests that CoQ_{10} is a safe and promising treatment for angina pectoris."

Another study, reported in 1984, looked at the effects of CoQ on angina when it is given intravenously instead of taken orally and came up with equally exciting results. In the Department of Cardiology at Komatsushima Red Cross Hospital, in Japan, eighteen angina sufferers were selected for the study. Twelve received daily 1.5 mg/kg intravenous infusions of CoQ for 7 days, while a control group of six patients received dummy placebo infusion. At the end of the trial the results were highly significant. When the CoQ group underwent treadmill tests 8 out of the 12 subjects were able to increase their exercise tolerance by one full stage (3 minutes per stage), while one patient actually managed an unexpected two stage jump. Three of the four remaining CoQ patients managed to increase their tolerance by at least 2 minutes. In summary, the measurement showed that the CoQ group averaged 4.55 minutes prior to treatment. By day 4 they reached an average of 6.45, and by day 7, 7.15 minutes. By comparison, the placebo group showed no significant improvements during the 7 day period.

Study leader Dr. Yoshikazu Hiasa reported, "The results of this study suggest that when CoQ_{10} is administered at high-dose levels to patients with effort angina pectoris, it helps the mitochondrial electron transport system to function smoothly so that the efficiency of oxygen utilization in heart muscle improves. CoQ_{10} is therefore considered to be an effective drug for the treatment of angina pectoris, having an essentially different mechanism of action compared to that of conventional drugs."

These are just two of many tests that have proven the effectiveness in helping angina sufferers. They were both trials of short duration and did not take into account how long-term CoQ might not only produce increasing heart performance but might also lead to dispensing with potent drugs like nitroglycerin altogether.

CHAPTER 7

.

Strengthening the Heart Without Exercise

Only one thing really strengthens the heart, exercise. It induces the heart to beat more vigorously, increasing the dynamic efficiency of pumping blood, oxygen circulation, and the strength of the heart muscle itself. But when dealing with the heart there's a fine line between safety and effect, especially at the very start of a new exercise regimen. It can be detrimental to initially push too far too fast—whether jogging, running, walking, or participating in an aerobic class or cardiovascular workshop.

While many people like to exercise, there are others who lead sedentary lives, never giving their hearts an opportunity to work out. These people's hearts would surely benefit from exercise if only they were more motivated. Now there are some interesting new studies showing that the heart's performance and strength can actually be improved safely without the duress of exercise. CoQ researchers have discovered an important link between exercise and increased concentrations of CoQ in the heart.

Previous studies in this book clearly revealed that CoQ can perform its energy boosting and protective benefits on the compromised heart. But it has also become clear from animal studies that endurance training not only strengthens the heart, but increases the quantity of essential CoQ in the heart tissues. The presence of additional CoQ is obviously a key to the heart's increased bioenergetic performance. Wouldn't it therefore be far easier if we could simply take supplemental CoQ to increase CoQ levels in the heart without all the strenuous exercise, and still have the same beneficial effect of improved cardiac energy and function? The following research indicates that this is possible.

Cardiac CoQ

Researchers at the University of Michigan developed a study to evaluate what changes may result in the levels of CoQ in cardiac tissue after a prolonged regular program of exercise and published their results in 1984. As their subjects they chose laboratory rats. For 6 months the animals were put on a rodent version of an athletic training program. A group of sedentary rats without training facilities were used as a control.

At the university's Laboratory of Chemical Biology, the exercise rats lived in mini health spas that were individually equipped with running wheels. The rats underwent enforced exercise for a portion of each day, which was gradually increased as their stamina evolved. And they were also allowed to exercise voluntarily. Interestingly, the rats voluntarily ran a distance of about 7 miles a day at the beginning of the program, mostly at night. Then as the enforced training increased from about 30 minutes to a standard 120 minutes a day, the rats eased off on their voluntary night running and cut it back to only about 2 miles a day. At the end of the 6 months trial the exercise rats were found to not only be fitter than the controls, but they were trimmer, with a mean body weight of 89 percent that of the sedentary rats.

The most significant factor was discovered after the animals' hearts were biopsied. Analysis of cardiac tissue revealed a substantial increase in CoQ when compared to the hearts of unexercised rats. The CoQ content of the whole heart jumped from an average factor of 198 to 270—an increase of 36 percent! And as if to confirm that the heart, and only the heart, had benefited, the CoQ levels in the liver, kidney, brain, and other muscles remained almost unchanged.

As a conclusion the researchers reported that increased CoQ concentration in the heart tissue resulted in greater mitochondrial density enabling them to function at much higher energy levels for longer periods of time with less stress on the heart. If CoQ was the key to greater cardiac energy, what would happen if supplemental CoQ was given to sedentary humans? This question was answered by researchers in Belgium.

Strengthen without Exercise

A team of scientists from the Free University of Brussels reported in 1981 that CoQ had illustrated tremendous beneficial potential for the hearts of patients with cardiac disease, but few, if any, experiments had been performed in order to evaluate the effect of CoQ upon the myocardial and muscular performance of young healthy subjects.

Team leader, Dr. J.H.P. Vanfraechem brought together six healthy but sedentary young men. The subjects had no organic heart disease and normal blood pressure. They might have best been described as regular "desk jockeys" who had no personal exercise or fitness programs. Their average age was 22-years-old: average weight, 159 lbs; and average height was 5 ft. 11 in. Before starting on CoQ therapy, all the subjects were tested using exercise bicycles to measure their normal cardiac outputs and endurance until exhaustion. They were then started on 60 mg of CoQ a day orally for the next 4 to 8 weeks.

When the results of their physiological testing at the end of the study was compared to their previous performances, there was little doubt from the new heart parameters that a beneficial improvement was evident. The myocardial contractility of the heart at under medium stress condition (this is classified as a heart rate of 170 or 170 HR) had improved by 12 percent after 4 weeks, and at maximal output by 28 percent. The Heather Index (measuring overall heart efficiency) showed an increase of 35 percent after just 4 weeks on CoQ therapy.

The researchers noted that after 4 weeks on CoQ the initial effects appeared to level out and maintain the benefits. The reason for this is likely to be that CoQ had reached the optimal point of its effectiveness in the heart tissue, and therefore remained at a constant increased level (this could be considered a natural safety factor) without accepting more CoQ than necessary. In essence, CoQ supplements had taken up the slack in existing lower CoQ levels and maintained it at optimum levels.

Reported Dr. Vanfraechem, ". . . the maximal exercise load was continually increased during the 8 weeks that our subjects were submitted to CoQ_{10} administration. But not only the max values were improved, but also a very important criteria, the work capacity at 170 HR."

A word of explanation is called for here. Most sedentary

people wouldn't be expected to benefit from a boost in their maximal cardiac output because it's highly unlikely that they would find themselves in a position to need it. But it is likely that they might get up to a heart rate of 170 during the course of their everyday lives by, for example, walking, running, or when under unusual physical stress.

Dr. Vanfraechem adds, ". . . at 170 HR, which represents 80 percent of max cardio-respiratory solicitation, the improvement is markedly present and this is important for sedentary people."

Possibly the most important point is not really how well CoQ improved performance at maximal exercise capacity (remember, these are subjects who wouldn't be exercising anyway), but what it did for the heart when the body was at rest, or in a normal sedentary state. There was no doubt it significantly improved heart function at rest. Some figures here will help to illustrate the beneficial effect. The average stroke volume of the heart was 61.3 at the start of the study and increased to 68.1 by its end. Average cardiac output showed initial values of 5.16 that were increased to 5.95. And the Heather Index improved from 15.2 to 16.3.

In conclusion, Dr. Vanfraechem states, "The results of 8 weeks Coenzyme Q_{10} administration upon sedentary subjects submitted at calibrated efforts, suggested that an optimal effect appeared upon the cardio-respiratory parameters after 4 weeks followed by a tendency to stabilization at the 8th week. However, concerning non-exhaustive values the improvements were noticeable until the 8th week and this is the most important fact for sedentary people."

It is clear from this study that CoQ can, and will, improve the function, performance, and energy efficiency of the otherwise healthy human heart, without having to resort to exercise. So, if a person is deskbound, doesn't exercise regularly, or is simply not a physically active individual, then CoQ would seem a sensible, effective, and safe way to improve the performance of the heart (and, in the long term, its potential life span) within the everyday needs that it will experience. Since moderate exercise has other beneficial medical effects, a combination with CoQ would appear to be the most desirable path to take.

It also follows that if a person is already pursuing an exercise or fitness program, CoQ could also benefit by giving the heart's energy potential a bioenergetic boost, possibly adding more stamina and enjoyment to the workouts. But, a few words of warning. This is one unique study. As in regular exercise to improve the performance of the heart, the secret is to take everything gradually and let the heart become attuned to its newly found potential. It is dangerous to overdo exercises which may put undue stress on the heart when it is not accustomed to it.

Do not be lulled into the false sense of security that supplements of a beneficial nutrient—one that can aid the heart's performance—will also protect it against abuse. One final point on CoQ's strengthening of the heart without exercise. Although the Belgian study holds out new hope for improving the hearts and lives of sedentary people, it does not report on the heart's status after the study was terminated. The study suggests that if CoQ supplements are discontinued the beneficial effects may be lost as the levels of CoQ return to their previous norm as supplied through regular nutrition and the body's own ability to provide the coenzyme.

However, it is known that CoQ is completely safe to take over the long term, so there should be no reservations about taking the nutrient as a supplement for extended periods of time, possibly for life.

CHAPTER 8

•

Reversing High Blood Pressure

High blood pressure—or hypertension—is not to be taken lightly. There's every good reason for it being known as the "silent killer." Over 40 million American adults are presently diagnosed as suffering from high blood pressure. And that figure is ultraconservative—the real problem may be as high as at least a third of the total population of the United States.

Latest statistics from the American Heart Association indicate that 31,500 people died as a direct result of high blood pressure in 1982. But, again, this number is conservative, and it does not take into account the hundreds of thousands of other deaths in which high blood pressure may have played a major role.

The Association's hypertension experts have recently revised the definition for high blood pressure, and this could mean that another 18 to 20 million people have the problem in addition to the original estimated 40 million.

The facts about high blood pressure are frightening. What's even more shocking is that very few people take it as a serious threat to health, or even know that they have it. If you want to know if you have high blood pressure, don't expect obvious symptoms. This disease gives nothing away, with no outward signs of its progress. Combine the previous facts with the lack of symptoms displayed by hypertension, and it's easy to see why medical professionals have dubbed it the silent killer.

There are, however, a myriad of drugs and drug combinations to fight high blood pressure. These are chemical preparations that also very often have unwanted side effects (these are listed individually by the manufacturers of each drug or can be found in the *Physician's Desk Reference*). In general these side effects include skin eruptions and other allergic reactions, changes in sleep and sexual patterns, and other symptoms from the central nervous system, such as dizziness. Even short-term loss of memory has been noted in users of certain antihypertensives. Changes of the gastrointestinal functions are also a problem. Another factor is that diuretics cannot be prescribed for patients with kidney damage. Yet another problem with antihypertensives is that side effects can be cumulative because once high blood pressure has been diagnosed, a drug regimen will usually follow for life.

For some people, blood pressure can be lowered by dietary and nutritional manipulation. But nobody has yet found a permanent cure for the disease, and possibly the biggest single reason for that is because medical science still doesn't know precisely what causes it.

Now there is new hope for sufferers of hypertension. There is a mounting body of evidence to show that CoQ can play a crucial role in regulating blood pressure.

What Is Hypertension?

Blood pressure is the force of blood against the walls of the 1.6 million miles of arteries and veins in the human body. This force is created by the heart as it pumps blood to the tiniest capillaries of the body. Small arteries, called arterioles, actually regulate the pressure of the blood by expanding and contracting. When they contract, the heart must pump harder to push the blood through. If blood pressure increases and remains elevated, the heart is forced to continue this extra, and unnecessary, work. And it is not a transient illness, but a potentially serious disease state.

An undeniable fact is that high blood pressure adds to the workload of the heart and arteries. And it's obvious that this may, in turn, affect or even trigger, the course of states like heart disease and stroke. Another problem occurs when the heart works under undue pressure for long periods of time: it tends to enlarge. A slightly enlarged heart may cope quite adequately, but a severely enlarged heart loses its functional capacity much like an overinflated balloon.

Hypertension also puts increased pressure on the vessel walls. The eventual result is that once they lose their elasticity, due to natural processes of aging, the increased blood pressure can cause ruptures.

What's the Cause?

High blood pressure is a biological puzzle. Its cause is unknown in 90 percent of the victims suffering from the disease. A remaining 10 percent can have the disease diagnosed as stemming from underlying problems, such as congenital defects of arterial vessels, kidney abnormalities, thyroid gland abnormalities, a tumor of the adrenal gland, but most importantly, the erratic regulation of blood pressure by the brain through the nervous system. In medical terms high blood pressure could be either *primary* (essential hypertension) or *secondary* (associated with other diseases).

How Do You Spot It?

In the majority of cases, high blood pressure will go unnoticed for years, unless it is spotted in a regular medical examination. The lack of obvious symptoms is the single cause of this. When a person feels good, looks good, and has no reason to suspect high blood pressure, there's very little likelihood that he will bother to have his blood pressure checked by a medical professional. Forget the commonly held myth that to suffer from high blood pressure you have to exhibit a ruddy complexion, a flushed face, or have dizzy spells. The silent killer may show absolutely no symptoms until it has already wreaked its havoc internally.

But there is a simple way to identify it. This is by measuring the pressure on the inside of a main artery. And when this test is performed in the physician's office it takes only minutes and is quite painless. Blood pressure is measured in two counts: first, the force-surge of the blood as the heart beats, called systolic pressure; and second, the pressure in the vessel, diastolic pressure, in between beats. These measurements are read as numbers. For example, 122 systolic, and 85 diastolic, will be referred to as having a blood pressure of 122 over 85, or 122/85. The diastolic pressure is considered as the more crucial of the two readings because it indicates the true pressure within the arteries rather than the force of the heartbeat. Both these measurements are recorded in millimeters (mm). This refers to the pressure needed to raise a column of mercury to a specific height. For example, 136 systolic would mean the pressure needed to raise the mercury to 136 mm on the scale attached to the apparatus being used to measure the blood pressure.

These measurements taken in millimeters (mm), are obtained by using a device called a sphygmomanometer, which is an inflatable rubber cuff with an attachment from which the pressure readings are taken. The cuff is placed around a person's arm and then inflated with air. This action squeezes against, and compresses, a large artery in the arm, momentarily stopping the blood flow.

As the air is released in the cuff the constriction is decreased and the blood begins to flow again. A person taking the reading will listen through a stethoscope until a pulse, or beat, becomes audible. This happens at the point the pressure from the heartbeat is able to once more open up the artery for circulation. If the pressure is high, the pulse sound may appear at, for example, 160. A pressure of 130 would be considered within normal limits.

The blood begins to course freely again as the pressure from the cuff is decreased on the artery. The pulse sound will disappear altogether when the pressure from the cuff equals the pressure inside the arterial wall. This is the diastolic pressure. A reading of 105 would be considered high, while a reading of 85 could be considered a normal range.

The simple fact is that the higher the numbers, the more difficult it is for the blood to flow.

What's Normal and What's Not

It used to be accepted that a reading of 160/90 was an indication of high blood pressure.

But due to medical advances, and our better understanding of the crucial role of high blood pressure in certain disease states, hypertension experts from the American Heart Association have revised their guidelines. The sensitivity of organs, specifically the heart, brain, and kidneys, to the effects of high blood pressure is now believed to be greater than previously thought.

The new definition of high blood pressure now includes anyone who displays a reading of 140/90 or more.

Here are the latest parameters for high blood pressure.

Systolic:
    Borderline—anything between 140 and 159, when coupled with a normal diastolic reading.

Diastolic:
  Normal—85 to 89
  Mild—90 to 104
  Moderate—105 to 114
  Severe—115 and over

It is obvious from these figures that the internal pressure in the arteries, the diastolic reading, is of prime importance, whereas the force of the heartbeat, the systolic reading, is less of a threat to health.

Lowering Pressure

The first line of attack against high blood pressure is through the use of diuretics—medications that rid the body of excess fluids and salt (sodium). Drugs, known as vasodilators, can widen narrowed blood vessels to reduce pressure, and others can prevent vessels from constricting. Another way to reduce hypertension is through dietary manipulation to reduce the intake of salt. In addition, overweight people can often simply reduce high blood pressure by losing a few excess pounds.

White Coat Hypertension

A curious phenomenon known as "white coat hypertension" is now being widely accepted by physicians—and blood pressure readings are being evaluated accordingly.

It happens in the presence of a physician, or other medical professionals, when they arrive to take blood pressure readings. The sight of a doctor can prompt an immediate boost in blood pressure. Although this is a common and unwanted effect, it is considered as a completely normal and natural stress reaction. In hospital studies and in physicians' offices, noticeable blood pressure elevations above the norm have been recorded.

Increases in systolic pressure of 20 units, and elevations as high as 5 and 10 on the diastolic scale, have been observed. While these discrepancies are small in themselves, they have the ability to push a person from normal to borderline or mild hypertensive—making him or her a candidate for medications that should not be required.

Many physicians are now taking the precaution of taking two readings; the first before any examination procedure, and the second a few minutes later when the person is more relaxed. Another way to avoid this effect is to have the person at risk from hypertension monitor his own pressure during normal everyday life, and then have the physician assess an average from the individual daily readings.

The CoQ Link

Because the cause of hypertension is still a biological mystery, it is not fully understood what role CoQ plays in blood pressure. It is known from animal and clinical trials that CoQ can indeed lower elevated blood pressure.

With the knowledge that CoQ is essential for bioenergetic functions, we might assume that the nutrient is in some way "repairing" or "adjusting" a reduced level of cellular energy metabolism that might act as a trigger for hypertension. In this case CoQ would be correcting a deficiency that could be considered a root cause of the problem.

It might be theorized that CoQ's beneficial effect could be in boosting the energy levels of tired and lackluster cells in arterial walls that have become prone to weakness and narrowing. With this action CoQ could be both correcting a deficiency and helping with protection against a result of hypertension. There may also even be a link between hypertension and the immune system.

From the studies described in the following section, it is clear that CoQ can play a beneficial role in reversing hypertension, exactly how it achieves this will no doubt be pinpointed in future research.

Animal Studies

Researchers in Japan discovered a connection between the high levels of sodium and potassium in the blood and tissues of hypertensive patients and deficiencies of CoQ. When CoQ was used as a treatment, the ratio of sodium and potassium decreased. This action was much like the beneficial effect seen when high blood pressure patients remove salt (sodium) from their diets.

Other CoQ researchers had surmised that the antihypertensive action of CoQ may rest in its ability to decrease the hypersensitivity of blood vessels to norepinephrine, a potent brain chemical which may play an instrumental role in hypertension.

In the early seventies a very distinct connection was observed between CoQ deficiencies and high blood pressure in humans. A deficiency of CoQ was noticed in leucocytes, the immune system's white cells, in blood samples taken from patients suffering from hypertension. Leucocytes are very sensitive to CoQ levels and are therefore good indicators of a deficiency state. This fascinating observation prompted the suggestion that a deficiency of CoQ levels might be of clinical significance in human hypertension.

Researchers at the University of Texas set about testing the theory on rats. The animals were split up into three groups, a first which acted as a control, a second in which hypertension was induced, and a third with artificially induced hypertension, plus CoQ supplements.

The systolic blood pressure was elevated in both groups two and three compared to the normal rats, but the group three CoQ-treated animals displayed significantly smaller elevations of blood pressure. After 6 weeks of study the rats were sacrificed and the results examined. The CoQ treated rats also showed no signs of heart enlargement due to the hypertension, while the hypertensive rats, without treatment, displayed bigger, and heavier, hearts. A report on the studies suggested, "Perhaps the hypertensive state increases the need for Coenzyme Q_{10} which is not fulfilled by increased biosynthesis but can be provided through treatment with Coenzyme Q_{10}."

And the report added, "It can be suggested that an increased deficiency of coenzyme Q in the hypertensive state is an undesirable condition for effective bioenergetics and particularly as required for ion transport including sodium. Correction of a deficiency of Coenzyme Q_{10} would surely be a desirable contribution to the control of hypertension."

A study conducted by the Japanese pharmaceutical firm, the Eisai Company, in Tokyo, was reported on in the *Journal of Pharmacology and Experimental Therapeutics* in 1974. What made this series of experiments so interesting was that the researchers also looked at how CoQ could affect the known causes of hypertension.

In one group of 42 rats the adrenal gland was chemically manipulated in an effort to induce hypertension. The animals were then divided into three groups of 14 rats each. One group was used as a control, while the second received 1 mg/kg (one milligram per kilogram of weight) of CoQ daily, and the third group 10 mg/kg. At the end of 6 weeks, 7 of the

12 control animals were found to have hypertension exceeding 160 in systolic blood pressure. There was no significant difference between the groups that received the low or high doses of CoQ—but only 3 rats in these two groups developed hypertension in excess of 160.

A second experiment utilized the chemical deoxycorticosterone acetate, commonly known as DCA, which is a potent inducer of hypertension in animal models. After DCA introduction, 30 rats were divided into three groups of ten. Once again, one remained as a control while the other two received either 1 mg or 10 mg of CoQ.

In the control group the blood pressures jumped to an average above 200. But after administration of CoQ, rats in the two therapeutic groups showed a reduction of blood pressures averaging some 40 mm. The researchers commented, "It was noteworthy after the termination of Q-10 administration, the blood pressure remained at the reduced levels for the remainder of the observation period."

Renal hypertension is another known cause of high blood pressure, and in this set of experiments by the same scientists, hypertension was induced in dogs by clamping the renal artery, and eventually removing the right kidney. Out of the ten dogs that underwent the procedure all developed high blood pressure. Six dogs (three with acute hypertension and three with chronic) were given 10 mg/kg of CoQ for 13 days and the remaining four acted as controls.

Before treatment with CoQ the levels of systolic blood pressure were in the range of 170 to 210 mm for all three groups. After the 7th day of antihypertensive CoQ treatment the average maximum drop in pressure was as high as 50 mm.

In a final experiment by these researchers, a special strain of rats was used. These animals had been specifically bred to display genetically inherited hypertension. A first test involved 36 animals aged 14 weeks old, which were divided into three groups. Two groups were treated with CoQ and it was observed that these rats had a delayed development of hypertension when compared to the untreated animals.

A second test was carried out on older animals. Among these rats, averaging 21 weeks old, the mean blood pressure was 190 mm. After 4 weeks of study, the average pressure built up (as expected) to 205 mm in 14 animals used as controls. But, incredibly, in 14 additional animals receiving CoQ, the blood pressure not only didn't rise any further, it actually decreased to an average of 183 mm. When CoQ therapy was canceled, their blood pressures went up to the levels of the control rats.

To further reinforce these studies the researchers carried out CoQ administration tests on healthy, normotensive (blood pressure within normal range) rats. The animals were given 1, 10, and even 100 mg of CoQ a day—and it had absolutely no effect on their blood pressures!

The researchers concluded, "Although the exact mechanism of antihypertensive action of Q_{10} remains to be elucidated, the experimental data suggest the possible clinical significance of Q_{10} for hypertensive disease of various etiologies."

Reversing Hypertension

When approaching CoQ from the human point of view, one thing that never fails to inspire great respect is its multifaceted role in many disease states. But this poses a slight problem. When looking at the benefit of CoQ in one particular state of ill health, how does one know that the beneficial effect was not the result of correcting an underlying deficiency from another undiagnosed problem?

Because hypertension is believed to play an important role as an underlying factor in a multitude of human ills, teams of researchers from Japan and Texas decided to determine first what CoQ levels could be expected in a normal healthy population.

This was a scientifically astute move. And it had a dual value. If CoQ similarities could be confirmed between two distant healthy populations, then it would follow that future research findings from one population would no doubt apply to the other. For example, there would be little reason to think that the results of studies involving CoQ and hypertensive patients in Japan would not apply to high blood pressure sufferers in the United States.

This enlightened approach was to initially confirm the ratios of CoQ in healthy populations on both sides of the world. Its object was to recognize any obvious parallels and, it was hoped, to confirm them.

Working independently during the mid-seventies the researchers from the Institute for Biochemical Research at the University of Texas and the Center for Adult Diseases, in Osaka, Japan, tested healthy groups of people to draw an assessment (by measuring blood content) of what levels of CoQ in the body could be considered as normal.

In Austin, the U.S. researchers reported that after examining dozens of healthy people, an average deficiency value of CoQ could be drawn for a general population. Not every healthy person can be expected to have 100 percent optimum amounts of CoQ available all the time, so it was not surprising that a small deficiency would be found in any given group of healthy adults. The mean deficiency of CoQ activity in the U.S. group was reported to be about 7 percent.

The Japanese researchers studied 65 healthy adults and their findings determined an average deficiency value of CoQ to be 7.6 percent; in other words, there was no significant difference between healthy CoQ levels in two populations on opposite sides of the world. This was extremely important because it set the baselines and ground rules for a major Japanese study among people suffering from hypertension.

The study to determine normal CoQ levels covered a wide variety of ages, from people in their thirties to subjects in their seventies. The Japanese results revealed:

Age	% Deficiency of CoQ
Under 39	6.9
40–49	9.8
50–59	6.2
Over 60	6.1

Average overall 7.6%

Then the researchers took 60 Japanese patients suffering from hypertension and subjected them to the same tests as the healthy population to determine their CoQ levels. The results among the hypertensive patients—who were suffering from high blood pressure only, without any complication from other diseases or states of ill health—clearly showed a much greater deficiency of CoQ.

Average readings for the hypertensive patients were a 22.6 percent deficiency of CoQ. This finding confirmed an extremely significant margin between CoQ in normotensive people and those suffering from high blood pressure.

The study went on to select a smaller group of the hypertension patients for therapy with CoQ. Seventeen subjects were involved and received daily dosages of 30 to 45 mg of CoQ for periods of 2 to 12 weeks.

Because of admitted inadequacies in some of the determinations performed during the study, the researchers chose to report on only four of these cases to illustrate the potential benefits of CoQ supplementation.

The following, Table I, illustrates their findings.

TABLE I

Effects of CoQ_{10} on the Blood Pressure of Patients with Essential Hypertension

| Patient | | Dose | Blood Pressure | | |
Age	Sex		Before (Highest)	With CoQ (Lowest)	After* (Highest)
23	F	30 mg/8 wks	208/130	150/90	186/126
		Before treatment average—176/112			
		During CoQ average —153/100			
		After CoQ average —175/122			
75	M	30 mg/16 wks	196/110	136/76	
		Before treatment average—187/99			
		During CoQ average —157/89			
71	M	45 mg/12 wks	190/108	168/88	208/108
		Before treatment average—190/94			
		During CoQ average —179/90			
		After CoQ average —202/102			
67	M	30 mg/4 wks	192/114	176/90	186/110
		Before treatment average—192/106			
		During CoQ average —178/94			
		After CoQ average —188/102			

*After means once CoQ was withdrawn

These test results show that addition of CoQ to the diet can help sufferers of hypertension reduce their high blood pressure—but the evidence does not indicate a cure for hypertension. The disease is believed to be vastly complicated with many systems of the body contributing to its cause.

The Japanese researchers believed that the bioenergetics of arterial walls was the suspected mode of CoQ's beneficial action in their test patients. Dr. Toru Yamagami, leader-author of the study, comments, "The direct cause of the maintenance of high blood pressure presumably is due to the contraction of the arterial wall. Accordingly, it is considered that the partial reduction of blood pressure in patients with essential hypertension when treated with CoQ_{10} may be due to the same mechanism. The contraction and relaxation of the arterial wall is presumably also dependent upon the efficient bioenergetics, as is skeletal muscle."

The researcher added, "It is presumably not in the best interests of the health of patients with essential hypertension to reduce their blood pressure by one of the commonly used antihypertensive drugs and allow their deficiency of Coenzyme Q_{10} to remain untreated."

This good sense approach recognizes that even though CoQ had a profound effect on reversing high blood pressure it did not totally halt the disease process or return it to normal. The nutrient appeared to be correcting some part of the processes that produce hypertension.

The benefits of handling hypertension with CoQ as an adjunct to traditional drug therapy were further echoed in follow-up research by Dr. Yamagami together with Dr. Karl Folkers, of the University of Texas. Once more, CoQ proved its benefit in a series of tests involving five patients. All showed deficiencies of CoQ in blood samples when first examined and before CoQ therapy was begun.

Only one of the patients showed no blood pressure improvement (in fact, a small increase), although his deficiency of CoQ was corrected almost immediately. But he was only on CoQ therapy for 8 days, and this tends to reaffirm that although a general deficiency of CoQ, as reflected in the blood, can be corrected quickly, it takes time for the coenzyme to work through and make an impact at the all-important cellular levels.

The following table (Table II) illustrates the results with the five hypertensive patients:

TABLE II

Effect of CoQ in Blood of Patients with CoQ Deficiencies and Hypertension

Patient Age	Sex	Dose	CoQ Deficiency % Before*	During†	Blood Pressure Before	During
35	M	75 mg/8 days	35	8	179/129	197/137
74	M	30 mg/5 mos	29	.78	176/94	148/86
49	F	75 mg/3 mos	20	4	186/97	153/84
45	F	75 mg/3 mos	30	12	166/106	143/93
69	M	30 mg/3 mos	40	19	193/114	179/106

*Before means prior to CoQ treatment
†During means while CoQ treatment was in progress

In four of these patients clear improvements were observable by a decrease in both systolic and diastolic blood pressure. Unlike the patient who showed no improvement, the patients who benefited took CoQ for a minimum of 3 months.

A report on the study by Dr. Yamagami and Dr. Folkers concluded, "Our interpretation of these data, both for reduction of blood pressure and for correction of CoQ_{10} deficiencies is based upon the concepts of bioenergetics since Coenzyme Q_{10} is indispensable to the bioenergetics which support life functions including blood pressure.

"CoQ_{10} is not properly considered as an antihypertensive drug, but rather as a vitamin-like substance existing naturally in human tissue. The 'antihypertensive' activity which CoQ_{10} appears to show may be the result of correcting a deficiency of it in bioenergetics. Such deficiency could contribute to mechanisms of hypertension."

One view of this study might be that the improvements were small, and it is quite fair to note that at least two of these patients would still be considered as candidates for conventional antihypertensive drug therapy. The obvious question then would be: Can CoQ be of value when it is combined with traditional antihypertensive medications?

The results of research at the University of Texas are illustrated in the next table, and this clearly shows the benefit of CoQ both as an adjunct to drug therapy and as an antihypertensive measure by itself.

In this table (Table III) you will notice that some patients were on medication and others were not. They all received 60 mg of CoQ a day over varying periods of time.

Table III

Reduction of Blood Pressure by Coenzyme Q_{10} in Patients with and without Conventional Drug Therapies

Sex	Age	Drugs	CoQ_{10} Dose Weeks	B.P. Before	B.P. After
M	50	X	60/12	134/96	113/84
M	51	X	60/12	132/95	124/86
M	60	X	60/5	166/93	142/82
M	36	X	60/9	139/91	128/83
M	43	Hg	60/5	177/103	164/100
M	39	X	60/5	150/92	138/88
F	69	X	60/12	206/97	164/79
M	44	X	60/11	190/143	166/117
M	66	X	60/15	155/116	132/105
F	62	X	60/12	188/80	175/78
M	65	X	60/13	244/98	193/85
F	73	Hd	60/16	161/97	141/78
F	50	Dy	60/16	166/98	137/84
F	58	Al	60/12	171/95	136/76
M	58	Lo	60/8	149/96	125/81
M	71	X	60/8	156/84	140/78

X = Untreated
Hg—Hygroton
Hd—Hydrochlorothiazide
Dy—Dyazide
Al—Aldactone
Lo—Lopressor and Hygroton

But the benefits of CoQ also take on a very different significance when it's remembered that only a slight elevation in blood pressure is needed to push a person over the safety barrier from the realm of normal, to the realm of high blood pressure.

For a person who is borderline, mild, or even moderate hypertensive, CoQ may be the only additional therapy needed to bring their pressures back to a normal range. Because of the need for extended treatment, in many cases an entire lifetime, the obvious benefit of CoQ is its absolute lack of side effects, unlike every other antihypertensive drug.

CHAPTER 9

.

CoQ Aiding Surgery

One of the most exciting recent discoveries of the seemingly never-ending beneficial powers of coenzyme Q_{10} is its ability to protect body functions and organs that find themselves under adverse conditions—as, for example, in surgery, and especially in major invasive surgeries like open heart.

Remember that CoQ's name is also ubiquinone: it is ubiquitous (occurs everywhere) in all life, and is essential to life. From that perspective CoQ is again examined for its beneficial effect in protecting tissues against the potentially adverse side effects of major surgery.

From its roots at the mitochondria levels, CoQ can therefore exert a mighty influence to reinforce the bioenergetics of damaged or ailing tissues, for example, the less than healthy tissue that might have to be subjected to the trauma of surgery.

Bypass Surgery

Coronary artery bypass surgery saves lives by adding canals that bypass the natural arterial rivers of the heart. A triple or quadruple heart bypass simply means that three or four transplanted vessels have been grafted onto a person's heart to divert the flow of blood around arteries which have been blocked by disease states.

Bypass surgery is not a very complicated procedure. But it does involve opening the chest, exposing the beating and living heart, and having to handle it during surgery. This, of course, is a traumatic process, and one which can be judged an invasion of potential severity to a heart that is already under great stress.

In bypass surgery a vein, usually from the leg, is totally

removed and one end is grafted into the heart's main artery. The other end is then sutured into the affected artery immediately beyond the area of obstruction. An uninterrupted supply of blood can now course freely through the implanted vein, bypassing the blockage, and into the healthy part of the artery where it can continue on to feed the previously endangered tissues being served by that artery.

Because the technique is relatively simple and the body does not reject the vein, being its own transplanted tissue, it has been hailed as a great success in combatting the effects of coronary artery disease like atherosclerosis. It has become popular in recent years, and now millions of bypass surgeries have been performed. But it is not without its critics, and it is not without a mortality risk.

Many cardiac specialists complain that surgeons have abused the technique, with literally hundreds of thousands of procedures being performed unnecessarily. And the other main criticism is that heart disease victims who have successfully undergone bypass surgery and have a new lease on life, often do little or nothing to change their life-styles to prevent the same type of blockage problems occurring in other cardiac arteries, or even in the newly transplanted vessels.

Surgeons in the Department of Thoracic-Cardiovascular Surgery at the Tokyo Medical University were well aware of the importance of myocardial protection to improve operative results and postoperative cardiac function. Indeed the bioenergetic health of the heart is considered critical to the potential success of the operation and the healing process.

A number of cardiac drugs had been used experimentally to prepare the heart for surgery and improve its chances of successful recovery. The university doctors, knowing of the proven bioenergetic effects of CoQ, began a study to test CoQ's abilities to improve the chances of the patient undergoing bypass surgery successfully.

Two inevitable problems have to be faced during surgery. The first is that the heart usually suffers periods of ischemia, and this lack of oxygenated blood flow to the tissues could inflict additional heart damage. The other problem is the occurrence of a myocardial infarction, the death of small areas of heart tissue due to prolonged ischemia. Previous tests of CoQ had shown that CoQ can protect against the hypoxic (reduced oxygen) effects of ischemia, and, by strengthening the bioenergetics of the heart, could also protect against infarct, the actual death of tissue.

The study, published in 1984, involved 42 patients scheduled to undergo bypass surgery. The protocol was to pretreat some patients with CoQ, and the controls would be patients who received no CoQ.

CoQ was given at random to 24 of the 42 patients through a drip infusion—5 mg of CoQ per kilogram of body weight— the night before surgery, and then again 2 hours prior to the bypass procedure.

The results showed that CoQ treated patients had stronger and more stable heart signs in the acute post operative period. By taking laboratory readings of certain blood chemical levels, which indicate damage to the heart, the researchers found that these were lower in the CoQ treated group. The researchers concluded that the most probable effect of CoQ was to act on the heart cells and their mitochondria, providing protection from ischemia during the operation.

Tokyo Medical University's Dr. Makoto Sunamori summed up, "CoQ treatment was found to result in improved and more stable postoperative hemodynamic conditions. These results suggest that the beneficial effect of CoQ on cardiac performance is related to myocardial cellular protection."

Cardiac Valve Replacement

This technique is another major invasive surgical technique with a high risk factor, especially among those already suffering from severe ill health. Cardiac valve implants are used to replace faulty or worn valves in the heart. The cardiac valves are strictly one-way mechanisms, allowing blood to flow only in one direction. Once a valve's function deteriorates, blood can back up and pool in the heart. The effect is a distressing lack of efficiency in the heart's pumping power, which can seriously compromise life.

Modern surgical techniques replace the faulty valves with synthetic plastic and metal ball-valves similar in design to the valve that might be seen at the end of a skin diver's snorkel. But during the procedure the heart has to be opened and its blood supply clamped off while the old valve is removed and a replacement sutured into place. When more than one artificial valve is needed the surgery can take many hours. Because of this the heart is at its most vulnerable. Even though

chilling methods and chemicals are used to preserve its biological integrity during surgery, the heart can still suffer.

One of the biggest fears facing cardiac surgeons is that even
when the organ is reconnected to its natural life-sustaining
blood supply it may not have the bioenergetic ability to start
pumping again. This is a constant life-threatening dilemma
that is usually overcome with inotropic (muscle contracting)
agents, like dopamine, which reenergize the organ. The heart
is literally being "jump" started.

Surgeons from the Division of Cardiovascular Surgery at
Kyushu University, Japan, began a study to test CoQ's
bioenergetic abilities to protect and boost the heart's potential
during major surgery. For over 6 years CoQ has been officially approved by the Japanese Ministry of Health and Wel-
fare as an inotropic agent for congestive heart failure.

Fifty patients requiring heart valve replacement were selected for study. They were randomly assigned to either a
group to be pretreated before surgery with CoQ or to a
control group, each consisting of 25 patients. The CoQ patients were administered 30 to 60 mg of the nutrient orally
for 6 days before surgery.

The surgery-protecting effect of CoQ was once more found to
be dramatic. All patients survived, but the CoQ group displayed
remarkably higher recovery rates. Among the group of 25 patients receiving CoQ, only 10 (or 40 percent) required inotropic
boosting when they were weaned off the cardiopulmonary
bypass machine. Of these 10 only 4 were considered severe.

In direct contrast 18 patients in the control group (or 72
percent) needed inotropic medication, and of these 12 were
classified as severe.

There was also a rather fascinating single case history. One
patient in the CoQ group, who had a total of 298 minutes of
operative time—the longest period for any patient in the study—
during which his aorta was clamped, required no heart boosting
at the end of surgery. This CoQ patient had not only undergone
triple-valve replacement, but a dacron patch had also been
sutured over a small rupture in the aortic artery—yet this
heart had bounced straight back without any apparent ill effects
from the surgery. These results were published in 1982 in
the American publication *The Annals of Thoracic Surgery*.

One of the Japanese team, Dr. Jiro Tanaka, confirmed,
"The incidence of severe low cardiac output state in Group 1
[CoQ] patients was significantly lower than in Group 2 pa-

tients, regardless of the duration of aortic cross-clamping. In Group 2, the percent of patients with severe low cardiac output state was more than twice that in Group 1 during the corresponding time periods."

Dr. Tanaka added, "The results of the present study suggest that preoperative administration of Coenzyme Q_{10} can increase the tolerance of human hearts to ischemia, as indicated by a significantly lower incidence of low cardiac output state following open-heart operation necessitating administration of considerable amounts of inotropic agent."

The focus of CoQ's bioenergetic abilities has been predominantly on the heart, and now its protective abilities are being vividly illustrated in heart surgery. The reason we are seeing CoQ introduced into the hospital ward and the operating room for the heart, and not for other forms of surgery at the moment, is simply because cardiac surgeons are the ones most familiar with the coenzyme's potential.

In witnessing the protective shield of CoQ in surgery involving the most vital of organs, these displays of effectiveness must surely raise questions about the possibility of benefits for the tissues of other organs—in transplant procedures, for example.

Transplants

Any natural nutrient that helps prevent the injury and death of tissue during cardiac surgery by boosting its bioenergetic capacity, its "survivability factor," must surely be worth further investigation in other surgical fields, especially in transplants.

One of the main obstacles to transplant surgery is the availability of a "fresh" donor organ. Methods can be used to preserve the integrity of the transplant organ, by chilling it, stabilizing it with chemical solutions, and rushing it into the operating room as soon as humanly and mechanically possible.

Because the vast majority of transplant organs come from the victims of accidental deaths, the organs first have to be removed and often transported to a medical institution which may be on the other side of the state, or even the country.

Knowing of CoQ's benefits in preventing the effects of ischemia in living tissue inside the body, wouldn't it be an incredible boon to transplantation if CoQ could do the same to protect organs once they had left the donor's body?

Livers are particularly sensitive to damage during transplantation, and, at the present time, a heart-beating cadaver is the only acceptable donor for a successful liver transplant. The breakthrough for organ transplantation utilizing the benefits of CoQ may not be far away if the latest studies using liver transplants in animal models are followed.

Researchers at Osaka University Medical School, in Japan, have successfully managed to transplant livers from dogs— without having to follow the normal restrictions of "instant" transplants from a body with a functioning heart. They were to achieve this only with the introduction of CoQ.

Research leader Dr. M. Monden reported in 1984, "At the present time, a heart-beating cadaver is the only donor for successful liver transplantation, since the liver is very sensitive to ischemic. Present restrictions to liver transplant would be reduced if greater use could be made of non-heart-beating cadavers as donors. Coenzyme Q_{10} (CoQ) has been reported to have protective effects on ischemic myocardium and recently on rat ischemic liver." Previous experiments during the late seventies at the Hiroshima University School of Medicine had revealed this fact.

Blood supplies to the livers of two groups of rats were clamped off for 90 minutes. None of the rats survived the ischemia in the first group. But in the second group with CoQ, 58 percent lived through the experiment.

The Osaka researchers conducted two separate experiments, the first to test out their CoQ transplant theories, and the second to try to determine how CoQ afforded its protection.

The first study utilized thirty experimental dogs as donors. Ten were used as "live" donors. The livers of ten more were removed after death and transplanted 30 minutes later. The third group of dogs were pretreated with CoQ just 60 minutes before they were sacrificed and their organs were also transplanted 30 minutes after death. The results were significantly clear-cut in favor of CoQ's benefits. Eight of the ten fresh liver transplants survived more than 6 days. Nine out of the ten cadaveric transplants in the second group perished within 24 hours. But in the cadaveric group with CoQ protection, six out of the ten survived longer than 3 days.

In the second study, ten dogs had artificial ischemia induced for 75 minutes by clamping off the blood supplies to their livers. A second group of eleven, all of whom were pretreated with CoQ, received the same procedure. None of the first ten animals survived more than 24 hours, but in the eleven member CoQ group seven survived for over 3 days "without any sign of sickness," reported the researchers.

But the interesting part of the experiment was discovering that CoQ worked at a cellular level by protecting and restoring the livers' bioenergetic functions. In the first group their ATP [cellular energy] levels decreased from 8.7 to 1.0 during the experiment and never recovered. However, in the CoQ group they dropped from 8.2 to 0.3 but rose to 4.0 after the blood supply was restored.

In a report the researchers deduced, "CoQ treatment is capable of enhancing hepatic [liver] ATP regeneration and keeping a high energy charge following reoxygenation. Seventy-five minutes of warm hepatic ischaemia was well tolerated by the dogs pretreated with CoQ. Enhanced ATP regeneration in the CoQ-treated dogs might be responsible for this cytoprotective [cell protection] effect."

There was no doubt from these experiments that CoQ protected the liver once it had been removed for transplantation, and clearly, once the liver's blood supply had been extinguished, the coenzyme shielded the organ's bioenergetic (ATP) abilities from deteriorating.

In the operating room for human liver transplantation, the ability to prolong the "life" of a fresh organ for even just a few minutes once it has been removed from the donor, can mean the difference between success and failure in surgery.

Artificial Organ Transplants—Protecting the Brain

The artificial heart is a wonderful breakthrough, not only as a full replacement for the human heart but as a stop-gap measure while a human donor is being found. But it has been plagued with problems. New research from France indicates that CoQ may play yet another crucial role, this time in making artificial heart transplants a safer and more viable procedure.

One of the obvious detrimental side effects to come to light after the limited number of artificial heart transplantations already performed is the high incidence of brain stroke complications. This appears to be a mechanical drawback that may weigh very heavily against the future of this type of artificial implant. The problem arises from blood clots which can clog minute vessels in the brain: this is called an embolism. In addition a blood vessel afflicted with artereosclerosis can rupture causing life-threatening complications. Both processes result in oxygen starvation. No matter how transient and short-lived these oxygen "outages" may be, they have a profound effect on the cells of the brain. We discussed earlier in this book just how supersensitive the brain cells are to lack of oxygen. In artificial heart transplants an inevitable side effect is strokes, which may, or may not, result in irreversible brain damage, such as mental and motor impairment.

Could CoQ once again offer the same protection against ischemia in brain cells as it does in others?

Dr. Jean Cahn of the Institute for Experimental Therapy and Clinical Research, in Montrouge, France, has shown that CoQ can also produce its benefits in the brain by protecting brain cells against the ravages of transient ischemia. At the moment this finding has only been observed in animals, but, as we have already witnessed, proof has to be shown to exist in animal models first.

Dr. Cahn's work with dogs, reported in 1981, set out to show that pretreatment with CoQ could diminish or abolish the neurological changes suffered during an artificially induced cerebral infarct—a stroke.

Fourteen dogs were used as controls, and six dogs were pretreated with CoQ orally for 2 days before the experimental procedure. The cerebral infarcts were induced by an injection of a chemical. Using sophisticated analysis of brain chemical components, Dr. Cahn was able to show that the CoQ group suffered significantly diminished ischemia and also swelling due to the induced injuries. The researcher had also witnessed the same effects of CoQ protection in artificially induced strokes in rats, which did not display any of the marked deficiencies in brain function normally associated with stroke trauma.

Dr. Cahn's studies may not only provide a new basis for a safer future in artificial heart transplants, but it may afford new protection in a whole host of surgical procedures involving the brain.

Another extremely important application of Dr. Cahn's research is the treatment of brain damaged patients (for example, victims of automobile accidents) with CoQ immediately on arrival at medical centers. This form of CoQ therapy can aid in preventing further damage to brain tissues already injured as a result of an accident and prevent additional damage during the trauma of brain surgery.

CHAPTER 10

•

CoQ and Adriamycin against Cancer

CoQ versus cancer: a once remarkable expectation that has now become a distinct reality. It wouldn't be considered imprudent to make a prediction at this point: The first clinical application of CoQ to be approved in the United States will be in an anticancer role.

Cancer is the second leading cause of all deaths in the United States. In 1984 alone there were an estimated 870,000 reported new cases of cancers, with the majority involving the digestive organs (colon and rectum), followed by the respiratory organs (lung), the genital organs (uterus in women, prostate in men), and the breast in women. Estimated annual deaths from cancer in recent years run to about 245,000 for males and just over 200,000 for females.

The role of CoQ in cancer therapy is not mere speculation. Our research at the New England Institute established that CoQ alone is effective in reducing incidence and mortality in experimental animals with induced tumors or leukemia. Furthermore, CoQ therapy boosts the beneficial effect of "classical" anticancer drugs. This is discussed in detail in Chapter 3. In an extension of our animal studies, Phase I clinical tests involving CoQ and cancer patients have been completed and accepted by the FDA. Phase II studies are under way in the United States and worldwide.

Many researchers are now discovering that CoQ can aid in the war on cancer by helping to prevent the highly toxic side effects of potent anticancer drugs. CoQ is again working its protective benefits, this time to shore up the defenses of cells in the body when they face injury, and possibly death, from the side effects of toxic chemicals. It's an unfortunate fact of life about many cancer chemotherapy treatments that they usually destroy healthy cells along with the tumors that they were aimed at.

An important point to consider when understanding cancer and cancer treatments, is that cancerous cells are not invaders from the outside. They do not enter our bodies like germs and viruses and then wreak havoc by making their new home inside us. Cancer cells are part of us. Tumors that have developed inside our bodies are as much a part of ourselves as a little finger, a toenail, a tongue, or even the heart itself. They are radical offsprings of cells that we have produced ourselves.

The difference is that these masses of cells follow none of the directions from the body's central blueprints. Cancer cells have wills of their own, they roam wherever they want, build in areas they're not allowed, and reproduce at the expense of other cells around them. A cancer grows unchecked because it doesn't recognize any of the body's preprogramed instructions for cellular reproduction; it continues to flourish as a cellular mass sucking in vital nutrients needed by surrounding healthy cells, gagging and strangling them, elbowing them out of the way, until it has commandeered control of all the locally available nutritional pathways and blood vessels.

When this runaway growth takes place in an organ, healthy cells, programed to perform the functions of the organ, are displaced by renegade cells which have no other object but to reproduce in a disorganized fashion. As the cancerous tumor takes over, the whole integrity of the organ begins to fall apart. Whatever valuable functions it produced previously are now being lost. The cancer has won control. Its unstoppable progression continues until the death of the organ and, ultimately, its owner.

Cancer can also spread uncontrolledly throughout the body. There's a natural transportation system of migrating cells, mainly through the blood and lymph system, which can present an unfortunate problem for the cancer victim.

Breakaway cells from a cancer tumor can enter the lymph and blood systems and wander to other parts of the body where they begin to breed new colonies of cancer cells to form more tumors. In medical terms this is called metastasis, and it is the most feared progression of the disease state for cancer victims who may have already had a primary tumor removed. The hope is that the disease has not already metastasized to other regions of the body.

Chemicals against Cancer

An attempt to stop tumor growth, and the process of metastasis, can be instigated early in the disease process by resorting to, among other things, chemical destruction of the cancer cells. Unfortunately chemotherapeutic action is nonspecific, and healthy cells are also sacrificed, though sometimes not immediately, as the drug toxicity spreads throughout the entire body.

An understanding of how chemotherapeutic drugs work is essential to being able to appreciate how CoQ can protect healthy cells. These drugs are essentially safe at low dosages, but as the dosages are increased, so is their toxicity and potential killing power for healthy tissue cells. There's an extremely fine line between a killing effect on tumor cells and the killing effect for normal cells. It is this narrow margin which makes these drugs dangerous as cancer fighters, because cancer cells are only slightly more susceptible to their toxic effects than healthy cells.

The therapeutic window is a small one to aim at when the oncologist has to recommend dosages of these anticancer drugs. A few grams too little and the drug will have little or no effect; a few grams too much and it will not only kill the cancer cells but healthy cells as well. The same problem is also seen by the radiologist who bombards tissue with radiation. He knows that cancer cells are slightly more prone to the killing effects of radiation, so he must measure his radiation blast to such a minute tolerance that it is deadly to the cancer while reasonably safe for surrounding healthy cells.

This problem can be appreciated by comparing an anticancer drug to a regular therapeutic drug. In the case of the regular drug, the optimal therapeutic dose could be 50 mg, and no toxic effects would be expected to be seen until you exceed at least ten times that dose, or, in this case, 500 mg. With cancer chemotherapeutic drugs a toxic effect occurs at the same level as the optimum therapeutic dose, and life-threatening side effects may develop with only double the dosage. Effectively administering anticancer drugs is a fine art.

But there's an additional problem. All those "safe" doses can build up to toxic levels over time as they are absorbed into other tissues in the body. And one of the areas of tissue particularly susceptible to the most common class of anticancer agents is the heart.

Buffering with CoQ

One of the most widely used classes of chemotherapeutic agents are anthracyclines. This class of compounds contains some of the most valuable antitumor agents. One of them, Adriamycin, has the most broad spectrum of activity of any available cancer killer. In fact, Adriamycin (a proprietary trade name) is such an effective cancer killer that patients, who years ago might have been expected to die, are living longer than ever. But there's a problem here—some patients in remission from cancer are now showing signs of heart disease that they never had. Medical researchers have discovered that some cancer patients are now developing toxicity from the long-term treatment with Adriamycin. It's long been known that the potent chemotherapeutic can also have a dilatory effect on the sensitive cells of the heart muscle.

Adriamycin toxicity has been noticed in 2 to 20 percent of patients receiving the drug. They exhibit myocardial lesions. These facts are causing grave concern. The incidence of heart failure is estimated at 15 to 20 percent—but only among those people who are considered as already displaying heart disease risk factors. Risk factors include being of an age greater than 70, having underlying valvular, coronary, or myocardial disease, and a history of hypertension. Otherwise, among the heart-healthy population, the risk factor from Adriamycin is only 2 percent.

An undeniable fact is that many cancer victims are older people who also have heart problems. And this is where CoQ can once more exhibit its potential lifesaving benefits.

As usual the first line of attack was to test for toxicity in animal models, and then prove what beneficial effects CoQ can contribute. Italian researcher Dr. Mario Ghione, of Farmitalia, in Milan, tested Adriamycin on the hearts of experimental rabbits and reported his finding in 1977. He discovered a significant depletion of CoQ in the heart after long-term administration of Adriamycin, and this corresponded well with the observations of increasing heart function failure due to the toxicity of the drug. But when additional supplies of CoQ were administered to hearts being depleted of CoQ by Adriamycin, a remarkable reversal process began to take place. The additional CoQ rapidly reversed the toxic effects of Adriamycin.

Researchers at the Federal Institute of Technology and the

University of Zurich, in Switzerland, also published findings in 1977 that demonstrated cardiotoxicity of Adriamycin in rats. And then rats were treated with both Adriamycin and CoQ together.

Team leader Dr. Gerhard Zbinden reported, "Adriamycin caused a significant widening of the QRS complex on the ECG [a heart monitor reading which shows serious malfunctioning of the heart]. Rats receiving CoQ_{10} and adriamcyin exhibited no significant change of the ECG [heart monitor]."

The Institute for Biomedical Research, University of Texas at Austin, also studied the effects of pretreating animals with CoQ before administering Adriamycin.

In two control studies, mice given Adriamycin had only 36 and 42 percent survival rates. But when two groups of mice were treated with CoQ for 4 consecutive days prior to Adriamycin introduction, the survival rate jumped to 80 and 86 percent.

The Institute's Dr. Alan B. Combs reported in 1981, "The diminution of the cardio and other toxicity of Adriamycin in cancer patients by prophylactic treatment with CoQ_{10} remains an important prospect."

Tests were also conducted in the seventies at Juntendo University, in Tokyo, to compare the protective effect of CoQ with two other drugs, nifedipine and propranolol, which were also suspected to aid in preventing the toxic effect of Adriamycin.

Rats were given large doses of Adriamycin to study the effect it exhibited on their hearts. Severe myocardial lesions resulted. But when the same dosages of the drug were given along with CoQ, or the drug nifedipine, there was a "reduction in both the incidence and the severity of the ADM [Adriamycin]-induced myocardial lesions," reported the researchers.

Scientists at the Japanese Tsukubu Research Laboratories found it very significant that Adriamycin's active role in killing cancer cells was the result of the drug's injuring the energy metabolism within the cell mitochondria. Knowing that CoQ plays an important role and also exerts a beneficial protective effect on the mitochondria respiratory (energy) chain, they concluded it may prevent the powerful damaging effect of Adriamycin on healthy cells.

Adriamycin was administered to guinea pigs in sufficient dosages to cause cardiac toxicity. Half the experimental animals received Adriamycin, and the other half were administered the drug after being presented with CoQ. The results: The expected damage to the mitochondrial energy function did not happen to the hearts of the CoQ treated guinea pigs! Their hearts' vital energy functions had been protected by CoQ. It was clear, at least in animal models, that CoQ had the ability to protect the heart from the ravages of this particularly toxic anticancer drug.

Knowing the protective value of CoQ, researchers at the Methodist Hospital in Indianapolis, Indiana, decided to investigate the potential of combining CoQ with Adriamycin treatments for patients with lung cancer.

Fourteen patients were divided into two groups of seven each. Group I received normal doses of Adriamycin, while Group II were administered Adriamycin plus 100 mg of CoQ orally per day. This group was also pretreated with CoQ for 3 to 5 days prior to starting on the potent anticancer drug.

The object of the study was to gradually increase the dosages of Adriamycin until a cardiotoxic clinical effect was observed. The heart's reaction to the dosages was constantly measured by impedance cardiography.

At the end of the study period the researchers were able to conclude that patients who had received Adriamycin plus CoQ were able to tolerate larger dosages of the drug with little or no changes in their heart functions. The control group, with Adriamycin alone, displayed expected heart problems, with decreases in all measured parameters, including cardiac output, stroke volume, and heart rate.

Dr. W. V. Judy reported in 1984, "This study demonstrates the therapeutic effectiveness of CoQ_{10} against Adriamycin-induced cardiotoxicity. Group II, treated with Adriamycin and CoQ_{10} received a significantly greater total accumulated dosage of Adriamycin without significant changes in cardiac hemodynamics or kinetics as measured by the electrical impedance method."

At the Queens Hospital Center-Long Island Jewish Medical Center, in New York, 11 patients with various cancers who were scheduled to receive Adriamycin therapy were also given CoQ.

Dr. Engracio P. Cortes reported in 1976 that the patients were treated with CoQ in doses of 50 mg orally each day at the start of Adriamycin treatment. He stated, "Preliminary results indicate that CoQ_{10} administration can prevent the early Adriamycin-induced cardiotoxicity."

In a follow-up study Dr. Cortes monitored eight cancer patients receiving Adriamycin who were given additional supplements of 50 mg of CoQ per day. The combined treatment resulted in a decreased incidence of cardiac dysfunction in six of the patients, and only marginal dysfunction in the remaining two. "CoQ_{10} was nontoxic and did not affect the antitumor activity or modify the ADM [Adriamycin]-induced bone marrow toxicity," added Dr. Cortes.

It indicated an intriguing possibility. By carefully manipulating the dosages of Adriamycin and CoQ together, the best of both worlds could be achieved.

In 1981 we described our studies which identified another side effect of Adriamycin. This was a powerful depression of the immune system—the same system that is so important in the body's fight against cancer. The reversal of this ill effect by CoQ_{10} is presented in Chapter 3 on the immune system.

More cancer researchers are now becoming aware of the prophylactic potential of CoQ as an adjunct to toxic cancer therapy. It makes sense to work hand in hand with an agent that can provide protection where the effect of chemotherapy is not wanted or needed. Extensive long-term clinical studies are needed. This will be the first clinical use of CoQ as a prescription drug in this country.

Meanwhile, individual researchers are able to chronicle cancer patients in remission who also happen to be participating in CoQ heart treatment studies that are not directed at alleviating chemotherapy toxicity.

One such case, described by Dr. Karl Folkers, involves a lung cancer patient who has been taking CoQ supplements together with Adriamycin for 5 years. During this period of combined treatment the patient was able to avoid symptoms of heart failure so often associated with long-term Adriamycin therapy. The patient, identified as R.G., started combined therapy when he was 49-years-old and for the next few years his dosages of CoQ were carefully manipulated to see if alternating them would have any bearing on the possible toxicity affect of Adriamycin.

Dr. Folkers reports that his cardiac efficiency was lower at 20 mg of CoQ a day than at 60 mg. When the dosage was increased to 100 mg there was no significant difference in the performance of the heart from when it was at 60 mg. But when the dosage was dropped back to 20 mg, his cardiac efficiency fell accordingly. It was decided to maintain him on 100 mg of CoQ a day.

Comments Dr. Folkers, "His cardiac output and stroke volume have been consistently elevated from the 17th month to the 60th month. As of October 1983, R.G. was still in remission after 5 years from lung cancer."

CHAPTER 11

.

Reversing Gum Disease

Periodontal disease is a scourge on our society. It accounts for more lost teeth in adulthood than any other dental problem. Gum disease will affect nine out of ten Americans within their lifetime, and one out of every four persons will lose all their teeth to periodontal disease by the time they reach age 60.

Even more disturbing is the fact that 32 million Americans have gum disease right now in such an advanced state that they will lose teeth if they don't receive immediate attention.

Periodontal disease doesn't just mean losing teeth. In its most serious forms it can cause facial disfigurement, abject pain, malnutrition from the inability to eat, and the social stigma resulting from the inability to retain acceptable standards of oral hygiene.

Millions of people undergo oral operations every year in a desperate effort to weed out the affected tissue with the surgeon's knife. For some others who are beyond surgical help, the only options are drugs, pain killers, and liquid foods. And it's because of the severity of the problem that many dentists are constantly frustrated when it comes to attempting cures for the rampant disease. But CoQ researchers are providing some beneficial good news for workers in the periodontal field. In case history after case history, "no hope" patients receiving CoQ as therapy have shown that not only is periodontal disease highly treatable, but its actually reversible.

How Does Periodontal Disease Form?

The process that accounts for 70 percent of all lost teeth starts out quite innocently as a buildup of bacteria into a colorless sticky film which constantly forms on the teeth. The bacteria is quite natural, and there's no real concern as long as it's continually removed by brushing or flossing.

This unwanted coating is called plaque, and it concentrates itself around the visual base of the teeth at the gum line, the start of the tooth's support system. Healthy gum tissue—called gingiva—and bone are all that anchor the tooth firmly in place.

If left in place the plaque bacteria make teeth surfaces their home while they digest the food that they keep being supplied with. Unfortunately, their by-products are not too savory, and they irritate the gums, which can become red, tender, and swollen and exhibit a tendency to bleed. When plaque is not removed it hardens into a deposit called calculus (or tartar), a form of cement which further reinforces the bacteria colony's hold on the tooth. Although calculus is inert, it makes the removal of new plaque even more difficult. A dentist or dental hygienist literally has to crack calculus off the teeth.

The tissue that attaches the gums to the teeth is eventually destroyed by the plaque's irritants and the gums begin to pull away from the teeth, forming pockets that then become filled with yet more plaque. This process moves down the tooth, steadily undermining all its foundations, and can eventually eat away at the jawbone itself. By now the tooth has become so loose that it either falls out or has to be removed by a dentist.

Meanwhile, the gum tissue has become diseased, and will continue to recede and die in a mess of infection and pain. At this point the gum may appear to have no energy to fight back against the disease process.

Latest research into periodontal disease shows it is not only a local problem. Bacteria-growing plaque, and especially their toxic products, enter the blood circulation and sensitize some of the cells of the immune system. This results in a decreased effectiveness of those immune cells, which may produce a generalized ill effect or locally aggravate the gum's redness and bleeding. Periodontal disease is now regarded as a generalized disease with a heavy involvement of the immune system.

And it is at even the most advanced stages of oral disaster that CoQ has been discovered to have greatly beneficial effects in re-energizing the gums and reversing the disease process locally and systemically through the immune system.

CoQ to the Rescue

As early as 1971 Dr. Karl Folkers, together with Dr. G. P. Littarru, were reporting that their research team had found a deficiency of CoQ in gingival tissue from patients with periodontal disease.

By 1973 Drs. T. Matsumura and Karl Folkers performed one of the first double-blind trials of CoQ versus regular periodontal treatments. All of the 24 patients involved had signs of serious destructive periodontal disease that had not responded to traditional oral hygiene methods, like extensive flossing and brushing.

Thirteen of the test subjects were treated with coenzyme Q—and the results were eye-opening. Nine of the patients responded dramatically to the natural coenzyme therapy plus regular periodontal care. In the placebo group of 11 subjects only 3 showed minor improvements during dental care plus placebo.

The researchers reported, "The therapeutic improvement of the patients with periodontal disease on treatment with coenzyme Q was better both in the number of improved patients and the degree of improvement than for the placebo group."

In 4 of the CoQ patients, symptoms of the disease had completely disappeared after an 8 week period of therapy. Once more, it was clear that CoQ was working its therapeutic benefits on yet another debilitating human illness.

In numerous studies between 1970 and 1975, scientists working with CoQ and gum disease came to these important conclusions: Since CoQ is an essential factor in cellular energy formation and is essential for the health of tissues, it would logically follow that increased availability of CoQ to deficient tissue should improve the bioenergetics of the tissue. With periodontal diseased tissue, it appeared that CoQ did exactly that. Then a series of remarkable studies was performed that involved U.S. servicemen.

One Researcher's Story

The research was spearheaded by Dr. Edward G. Wilkinson, and his staff of periodontists at the Wilford Hall U.S. Air Force Medical Center, and later at the Department of Periodontics at the David Grant USAF Medical Center on the Travis Air Force Base in California. As related in the Introduction of this book, Dr. Wilkinson was extremely skeptical of the claims he'd heard that CoQ could actually reverse periodontal disease.

An attitude like this was hardly surprising as Dr. Wilkinson, like many other dentists, was aware of the difficulties of halting the nonstop progression of the disease once it had reached severe stages. Usually the only option available was surgical removal of the diseased tissue.

Dr. Wilkinson and his team started their research by taking tissue samples from over 120 dental patients with periodontal disease, which confirmed a marked deficiency of CoQ_{10} in diseased gum tissue.

The following table illustrates the findings in 22 patients with obvious periodontal disease, and vividly shows obvious deficiencies in the percentage of CoQ activity in diseased gingival tissue extracted from their mouths.

TABLE I

Percentage Deficiencies of CoQ_{10} in Gingival Tissue of Patients with Obvious Periodontal Disease

Age	Sex	Systemic Condition	% Deficiency of CoQ_{10} Activity
34	F	Excess nervous	51
37	F	Iron Def. Anemia	—
36	F	Gastric Problems	23
36	F	Bruises Easily	30
54	M	Stomach Ulcer	12
41	M	No Med History	57
41	M	No Med H.	53
53	M	No Med H.	58
41	M	No Med H.	8
64	F	No Med H.	17
42	M	No Med H.	48
42	M	No Med H.	51
45	F	Excess Nervous	54
45	F	Drug Sensitivity	54
52	F	No Med H.	—
32	F	No Med H.	50
42	M	No Med H.	29
53	M	No Med H.	23
29	F	No Med H.	43
51	M	No Med H.	50
51	M	Coronary Condition	54
49	M	No Med H.	52

The next step was a follow-up study to take samples of both diseased and healthy tissue from the same mouths and compare them. The results could not be ignored. Healthy tissue taken from patients' mouths was not deficient in CoQ_{10}, while diseased tissue extracted from the same gums was.

This finding spurred on the dental researchers to conduct a double-blind trial where some periodontal patients were on daily regimens of oral CoQ supplements of 75 mg a day, while others were given placebo or none at all. The results were measured by gum pocket depth. This measurement is performed in the same way a dentist assesses the health of the gums, with a simple probe which is inserted between the tooth and the gums and measures the depth to which it can sink. Patients were also rated overall for gingival health, and assigned numeric values. After the experiment the results were assessed by five independent researchers.

In the following table of six sample patients, the pocket depths are clearly reduced after CoQ treatment (see Table II). A second table, Table III, illustrates periodontal scores for eight patients.

TABLE II
Periodontal Scores by Pocket Depth

Patient	Before CoQ Administration Average	After CoQ Administration Average
1	3.55 mm	1.91 mm
2	3.68	2.81
3	3.11	2.84
4	3.82	3.16
5	2.27	2.14
6	3.12	2.51

"What was very obvious was that when the researchers evaluated the results on a blind basis they were easily able to pick out the patients who had taken CoQ_{10}, and those who hadn't. There was a beneficial difference that was clearly visible," says Dr. Wilkinson.

In one study, which involved eight periodontal patients, whose conditions were serious enough for them to be already considered for surgery, dramatic improvements were recorded after just days on CoQ therapy at a dose of 50 mg a day.

TABLE III

Periodontal Scores by Pocket Depth

Patient	Before CoQ	After CoQ
1	1.85 mm	1.20 mm
2	1.45	1.00
3	1.20	1.05
4	2.15	1.55
5	1.85	1.65
6	1.75	1.15
7	1.25	1.15
8	1.65	1.15
	Av. 1.64	Av. 1.23

What impressed the scientists was that not only did the disease appear to have been stopped, but an incredible rate of healing was now being observed. One of the things not expected to be seen in diseased tissue is spontaneous healing; if anything, wounds inflicted on the tissue will get worse. But (as an illustration of CoQ's effectiveness) the surgeon who had performed biopsies to remove diseased tissue for analysis at the start of the experiment, was amazed to discover that his original biopsy sites were difficult to locate after just 5 to 7 days into the study. A report on the study referred to this phenomenon as "extraordinary healing"—which was further defined as "tissue healing in five days which would ordinarily be expected to heal in ten to fifteen days."

The results were so impressive that the USAF periodontists had before-and-after photographs of their patients examined by researchers from other fields of dentistry, and then even called in civilian dentists to review their findings.

The official report states, "A review of 2x2 transparencies taken during the course of the study demonstrated extraordinary healing. The evaluations of healing were made by the periodontal staff and by the staff of other dental disciplines. A civilian group of dentists, who had no information concerning this study, also evaluated the 2x2 transparencies and the combined opinions of these eight dentists supported the interpretation of improved healing."

Dr. Wilkinson's studies were also reviewed and verified by Dr. Karl Folkers. Comments Dr. Wilkinson, "What we were witnessing was, for lack of a more accurate medical phrase, not just a therapeutic treatment to alleviate symptoms, but a reversal of the disease state in some cases and a regrowth of healthy tissue."

He explains further, "Coenzyme Q_{10} is essential for every person to live. Without the presence of it the essential healthy functioning of the cells break down. There is no energy in the cell, in a very real sense it is dying. And this is what we see in periodontal disease. We see a lot of dead cells and inflammation of the connective tissues.

"It appears that most people have an adequate supply of CoQ_{10}, but some people don't seem to be able to assimilate it as well as others. Periodontal tissues are deficient in CoQ_{10} when they are diseased, and appear to require more CoQ_{10} to heal.

"I believe persons suffering from periodontal disease could benefit from Coenzyme Q_{10} as an adjunct to routine periodontal therapy."

Further Studies from Japan

Studies in Japan had also begun confirming CoQ's ability to reverse periodontal disease. Knowing of CoQ's crucial role in bioenergetics, the Japanese scientists also drew the conclusion that CoQ enabled the disease process in the gums to be reversed toward a healthier cellular state, which also promoted rapid healing.

From the Department of Periodontics at Hiroshima University School of Dentistry came a 12 week double-blind study, reported in 1981, in which an impressively large number of patients suffering from periodontal disease were followed. The average age of these patients was 42 years, and none of them had any other significant medical problems. The dentists examined the patients and recorded the changes of five clinical symptoms: gingival redness, swelling, pus discharge, tooth mobility, and depth of the periodontal pocket.

After examination each patient was given either a capsule of CoQ or a placebo. The daily dosage of CoQ was 60 mg, with each patient instructed to take one 20 mg capsule after meals. During the first 4 weeks patients were given only the CoQ or the placebo without any local treatment. The same therapy was continued for the next 8 weeks with the addition of periodontal treatments, which included scaling and instructions on tooth brushing. All the patients were thoroughly examined during the 4th and 12th week of the study. At the end of the research 49 patients had completed the study, 20 of them having received CoQ, and 29 the placebo. Again, the beneficial results of CoQ administration were unquestionable. The scientists reported, "Pus discharge and tooth mobility in the CoQ group showed statistically significant improvement in Exam. II [4 weeks] unlike in the placebo group. In tooth mobility the mean score in the CoQ group was a significantly lower value than the placebo group in [both] Exam. II and III. In addition, the average significant pocket depth in the CoQ group was also shown to be significantly shallower than that of the placebo group." And they concluded, "In this study these chronic conditions were improved during 4 weeks of oral administration of CoQ_{10} without any local treatment. It might be said that CoQ_{10} [alone] improves the chronic status of periodontal disease."

Numerous other studies in Japan have since confirmed the effectiveness of CoQ in the treatment of periodontal disease. But nothing illustrates the point better than actual case histories.

Selected Case Histories

The first two of the following dramatic case histories were related directly by Dr. Edward Wilkinson. The second two are from the files of his brother, Dr. Raymond F. Wilkinson, a former USAF dentist and a CoQ researcher.

Case I. Female patient, aged in her seventies. Diagnosis: desquamative gingivitis.
Dr. Wilkinson reported,

Desquamative gingivitis is an extremely severe form of gum disease. You have to understand that we don't even know what causes this type of oral disease, and there are no cures. I told this woman the sad story that we couldn't do anything for her. Her mouth was a mess, she couldn't even eat because she was in so much pain. She had run the gammet of traditional therapy without any apparent success. She was, I hated to admit, a no hope case. Nevertheless, I decided to try her on 75 milligrams of CoQ_{10} a day. Within two or three days the pain had subsided and she was eating again. The

initial improvement was dramatic. I kept her on CoQ
and symptoms of the disease began to greatly diminish.
It is unknown if the therapy actually "cured" the disease
state. But the fact still stands that she became healthier,
happier, and was able to return to a normal lifestyle.

Case II. Female patient, aged in her sixties. Diagnosis:
severe periodontal disease.
Reported Dr. Wilkinson,

> The condition of this patient was amongst the worst I
> have ever seen. This lady was diseased throughout the
> mouth and into the mucous membranes of her nose and
> throat. It was a pitiful sight. She was totally unable to
> eat, and was in severe pain and discomfort. She was
> given 75 mg of CoQ per day and received standard
> periodontal treatment. The prognosis for her condition
> was very poor, it was seriously advanced. But within two
> weeks of starting CoQ therapy she was eating again. Her
> overall condition began to markedly improve.

In reviewing these cases Dr. Wilkinson commented, "What
is interesting about these two subjects is that they were
literally no hope cases who went on to live pretty much
normal lives thanks to the simple addition of supplemental
CoQ to their diets. There were still signs of the disease
states, but the excruciating symptoms were greatly reduced
or reversed. Even if the disease itself could not be cured, the
agony of the affliction was relieved—and that can be considered as truly beneficial therapy."

Case III. Male patient, aged 47-years-old. Diagnosis: advanced gingivitis.
Patient's chief complaint was raw, highly inflamed gingiva
having a burning sensation. Biopsy showed massive chronic
inflammation of the gum cells and a tentative diagnosis of
gingivosis (desquamative gingivitis) was made. The patient
was unable to brush or floss his teeth because of the extreme
pain. He was put on a treatment of corticosteroids (a valuable
therapy, but with unwanted side effects, especially after extended treatment) and experienced some relief from pain but
the inflammation still continued. After almost 3 years of treatment without improvement, the patient was put on 30 mg of

CoQ_{10} per day. Within one week the patient experienced relief from pain enabling him to brush his teeth and the inflammation subsided. After 6 months the experimental CoQ_{10} therapy was discontinued. Within 4 days the patient experienced pain in toothbrushing, and it gradually worsened. Within 2 weeks the inflammation had returned. After 1 month the Coenzyme Q_{10} therapy was reinstated. The pain disappeared almost immediately and the swelling disappeared. The patient's situation remained stable on 30 milligrams of Coenzyme Q_{10} a day.

Case IV. Male patient, aged 34. Diagnosis: benign mucous membrane pemphigoid.

Patient's chief complaint was that of painful, reddened gingiva that he had had for approximately 2 years. Clinical examination revealed a generalized, acute inflammation and diffuse redness of the attached and marginal gingiva. After biopsy a diagnosis of benign mucous membrane pemphigoid was established. In January he began receiving 60 mg of Coenzyme Q_{10} per day. The most subjective symptom of pain was greatly reduced during the first month of therapy. The redness of the attached gingiva did not change during the first month. However, during the following months the erythema gradually was diminished. The patient is continuing this course of treatment.

These four case histories involved persons with periodontal disease who would have been looked upon as "no hope" cases by most dental professionals. Their prognosis might have been continued deterioration of the oral tissues process which were literally rotting in their mouths. Therapy would more than likely have been massive doses of antibiotics and pain-killers, combined with what little oral hygiene they were able to perform, given the painful circumstances. The treatment scenarios would not have been helping to effect a cure at the root of the problems.

CoQ's role in all four patients appears to be quite clear—it was somehow providing renewed life and vigor to the diseased gums, and thereby affording them a means to overcome, and reverse, the rampant disease state.

CHAPTER 12

·

Weight Loss through CoQ

The only safe and effective way to lose weight is through dietary manipulation. Excessive weight is produced according to an elemental equation: more calories consumed than required by energy-demands equals fat. And the equation to lose weight is equally simple: fewer calories consumed than necessary for energy requirements equals a reduction of fat.

Millions of dollars are spent each year on weight loss programs, and with all the diet plans, books, magazines, and even video cassettes offering the "ultimate" in weight reduction, it's hard to pick the one that might be the right choice for the individual.

Then there are the fad diets, which may be effective in the short term but they can be downright dangerous to health. Anybody can lose pounds a day eating only grapefruits, or grapefruit pills with accompanying tiny amounts of food. Weight loss will also be achieved in the same manner by eating only cucumbers, cauliflower, watermelons, apples, pumpkins, or even potatoes. If only small amounts of any foods are ingested each day, the result is bound to be weight reduction.

The problem with these types of medically unapproved dietary regimens is that they often do deliver what they promise in sudden weight loss, but at the expense of putting undue stress on the natural metabolism, the organ systems, and, essentially, overall good health. This weight loss is often impossible to retain when the dieters return to their previous eating habits. The important thing any dieter should ask is, Am I getting enough of the essential nutrients to sustain the ongoing life processes within my body? And the answer, with fad diets, is most probably, no. That's why they are so dangerous to health.

Foods supply calories. Caloric content is the heat, or energy, released from any compound. Calories from foods are units of "heat" which the body utilizes to convert to energy. When the body has sufficient calories to maintain life, it stores the remainder already ingested.

The fat we observe on the human body serves a very useful purpose, it is the warehouse for energy storage. The body is programmed not to waste its sources of energy, so it therefore makes deposits in what is referred to as fatty tissues. The problem of obesity occurs when the body is constantly overwhelmed with too much of the energy sources. The fat supplies will begin to grow if they are not converted to energy.

The best way to lose excess weight is through a combination of reduced caloric intake and increased energy demand over and above the intake levels: less food and more exercise. The body now has to turn to its fat reserves to supply the additional energy necessary for life.

Once the overweight person has reached a satisfactory weight goal, it is often difficult to maintain unless their new nutritional life-style supplies only enough calories to satisfy present energy demands. That is why a maintenance program of eating (with more calories than in the diet, but less than in the previous eating habits) is most important.

But how come some people can eat all they want and never get fat? This is a matter of individual metabolism; the energy equations between human bodies differ. Some people have overactive metabolisms that burn up as many calories as they wish to ingest, others have slower metabolisms that require less calories to perform efficiently. The ideal diet aid would be a mechanism that speeds up the sluggish metabolism, but without damaging the rest of the body.

CoQ may have this capability. A deficiency of CoQ could act to slow down the metabolism, while adequate CoQ levels regulate the effective "burning" of calories to produce energy. To be fair, this action of CoQ has not been entirely proven yet. More research needs to be conducted to further verify its effect on weight loss and weight management. Yet it surely does make sense that a crucial component of bioenergetics could play a key role in the mobilization and utilization of excess supplies of fat. Anything with the ability to speed up or make the metabolism of energy production more efficient, has to be a potential fat burner.

Most significant in the following research is this one fact: it appears that some people who are unable to burn up fat efficiently and stay within "normal" weight parameters, have a noticeable deficiency of CoQ!

CoQ Versus Obesity

Excess fat is not just cosmetically undesirable, it is a danger to health. Adult obesity is associated with a number of medical complications, such as coronary heart disease, artereosclerosis, hypertension, and many other metabolic disturbances.

Researchers in the department of Endocrinology, Metabolism, and Nutrition at the University of Antwerp, in Belgium, had noted CoQ's important role in benefiting the aforementioned conditions, and wondered if the energetic coenzyme might indeed play a role in obesity.

They noted in a report published in 1984 that recent studies in laboratory animals had revealed the existence of thermogenic active "brown adipose tissue"—or BAT, for short. In contrast to white adipose (fat) tissue, BAT was characterized by high amounts of mitochondria, responsible for cell respiration or thermogenesis. BAT, it could be said, is the tissue containing the powerhouse of stored energy.

Utilization of these stores, or thermogenesis, can be measured in increased oxygen consumption or heat production (a by-product of all energy is heat). Active thermogenesis prevents the onset of obesity—even in animals with elevated caloric intake. Humans with a family history of obesity have a thermogenic response to food that is only half that of a lean control group.

Human production of energy from food is much like a furnace. Somehow in obese people the furnace either doesn't get ignited at the right time or it doesn't burn at peak efficiency. Continued deliveries of fuel supplies therefore build up, even though they are not needed or wanted. Could CoQ hold a key to unlock this biological furnace?

Dr. Luc Van Gaal and his Belgian colleagues studied 27 obese subjects and found that their CoQ levels ranged between 0.48 and 0.84, or an average value of 0.62. It is generally recognized that the cutoff point for CoQ deficiency is .65; therefore as a single group they were deficient in CoQ. As it so happened, 14 of the 27 obese patients (or 51.8 percent) fell into a CoQ deficient category as single subjects.

Nine subjects, average age 37 years, were then selected for further clinical trials and divided into two research groups. Group A numbered five individuals who were deficient in CoQ, and Group B, four individuals who exhibited CoQ levels above the deficiency cutoff line. The two groups received similar controlled diets with balanced nutrition for an initial period of 9 weeks, and all individuals also received 100 mg of CoQ daily.

There was little to choose from between the two groups in total body weight; Group A was slightly heavier, averaging 242 lb, while Group B's mean weight was 228 lb.

At the end of the 9 weeks the low CoQ subjects, Group A, now with the benefit of added CoQ to their diets, managed to shed an average of 29.7 lb, while Group B could only manage an average of 12.7 lb. By the end of 3 months Group A had lost a respectable average of 37 lb, or 16.6 percent of their total body weight.

Dr. Van Gaal reported, "At this exploratory stage of the study, it may be presumed that very obese patients have approximately a 50 percent Q_{10} deficiency.

"It looks possible that correcting significant deficiencies of Q_{10} in obese patients might improve lipid metabolism and contribute to the metabolic or cellular control of body weight, although it is evident that many other aspects will be involved in obesity. On the basis of blood levels, the results of this exploratory study seem rather remarkable and encouraging."

Clearly CoQ is not a panacea for all weight problems, but it certainly holds out new hope where a natural reason for unwanted and unexpected weight gain cannot be found. The first avenue of attack could be to check the body's levels of CoQ.

In this study the obvious fact remains that people who were deficient in CoQ were able to shed more pounds when their CoQ levels were boosted than overweight people who had no CoQ deficiency. And remember that they were all following the same dietary guidelines. It could be assumed that the overweight problem for subjects with no CoQ deficiency might be attributed to other factors.

When a CoQ deficiency was discovered, and when that deficiency was corrected and the overweight subjects then began to lose weight, it could be assumed that the problem might have rested with some inability to utilize their energy-burning capacities at peak performance. Did CoQ provide the spark that lit the internal energy furnace and regulated it to now burn calories efficiently? Because the researchers in this study took a random sample of obese subjects, could it be assumed that over half of all overweight people may be suffering from a CoQ deficiency? This is likely, but it has yet to be proven in larger samplings.

But if this hypothesis is so, it then leads us to the conclusion that over half the sufferers of overweight conditions might be able to lose weight exceedingly simply—with the easy addition of CoQ supplements to their normal dietary regimen and nothing more life-style shattering than sensible nutrition without resorting to crash diets. For some over-weight people, CoQ may turn out to be the "ultimate," no-side-effect, diet pill of the future.

CHAPTER 13

.

Nutrition and CoQ Availability

CoQ, like vitamins and minerals, occurs naturally in many of our foods. But like these other important nutrients, it faces a similar problem—being "destroyed" before it reaches the dining table. In the average American diet, food quantity is no problem, but food quality is.

By the time foods have been picked, processed, packaged, dispatched, delivered, and displayed, many of these foods we take for granted as good sources of nutrition bear little of their original vitamin and mineral contents, and this, too, may apply to CoQ.

The problem of "missing" nutrients is more common among the canned, preformed, and prepackaged produce that we find on the supermarket shelves, especially with processed meats, fruits, and vegetables. For example, it may look like a can of asparagus, it may even taste like asparagus (or what we have grown to accept as the taste of asparagus), but, overall, the green vegetable fiber in its protective liquid is no more like fresh-picked asparagus than stewed celery.

The contents of processed foods will be wholesome and digestible—the processing has made sure of that—but the main body of healthful vitamins and minerals originally contained in the plant and animal products have long since departed due to the miracle of extending shelf life through food technology.

Other factors that can be detrimental to food quality include:

• Forced ripening of fruits with gas reduces nutritional value. Premature ripening produces a fruit that will cosmetically appear to be a mature product, but because it is not fully matured it lacks a fully developed nutritional content.

• Extended storage reduces nutritional values.

• Cooking destroys much of the nutritional value of many foods, especially vegetables.

But today some foods, especially cereals, are "fortified" with additions of vitamins and minerals. This certainly can help to compensate for the loss of vitamins A, C, E, and the Bs, or D in milk, for example, but unfortunately it does nothing to ensure our supplies of the CoQs.

Vitamins, Minerals, and CoQ

The previous observation on how foodstuffs lose their value before reaching the dinner table serves to illustrate just how transient essential nutrient content in foods can be. The good news, however, is that our most abundant supplies of CoQ_{10} come from animal tissues such as beef, pork and chicken, or fish, most of which are purchased "fresh" in the food stores without having gone through a processing phase.

It is the fragile chemical bonds that hold together essential nutrients (like the vitamins and CoQ) which make them so susceptible to "returning" to their original chemical elements. Understanding this may help the reader to realize why, although there is variety and quantity in the American diet, it can lack severely in quality.

A fact of all death, whether plant or animal, is that once life is extinguished, certain chemical changes take place within the organism that start to destroy its original chemical structures. Animals and plants compose chemically all their lives, and after death they start to decompose almost immediately, although at first this is at a microscopic molecular level and would be imperceptible to our vision or taste. Chemicals that were once held in check by the life process now take over, breaking valuable molecular bonds that formed the essential nutrients. As the elements continue to return to their basic forms, it's easy to see that all the valuable chemistry that went into creating nutritious combinations is beginning to quite literally fall apart.

Vegetables can lose up to 70 and 80 percent of their original vitamins and minerals within a day or so of being picked. The same process also applies to animal products, although refrigeration and chemical preservatives, for example salt, can slow this down appreciably.

A well-balanced diet that includes the essential vitamins

and minerals is of paramount importance to our overall health and well-being. "Well-balanced" is the operative phrase here. It won't do any good to eat mountains of a few single foods, like French fries, hamburgers, and cookies because, although they may supply quantity in calories, they will not provide quality and variety in nutrients.

There is a nutritional school of thought, however, that believes it is virtually impossible to receive the necessary amounts of vitamins and minerals through the average American diet alone. This is a source of controversy among nutritionists, with about 40 percent in favor of taking vitamin and mineral supplements in addition to the regular diet. The one obvious fact the pro-vitamin-supplement school always cites is the almost impossible task of keeping track of how much of the essential vitamins and minerals really do still exist in the product by the time it has reached the eating table.

The boom in the vitamin and food supplements industry has tried to fill this nutritional gap. Vitamin, mineral, or indeed CoQ supplements do not take the place of foods. Foods supply many other complex compounds that are also essential to life. Supplements are the nutrients once they have been isolated or synthesized and put into a form in which they will not lose significant amounts of their individual chemical integrity.

It is not the authors' intention to judge whether the average American food intake is adequate or to recommend taking supplements as a safeguard if it isn't, but rather to promote an awareness of food quality. The main concern in this chapter is to provide pointers that will help to ensure good nutrition, which in turn will further help to provide adequate supplies of CoQ and enhance its beneficial actions within the body. Human nutrition is, after all, an affair of complements— many different chemical combinations working hand in hand to complement and enhance each other's actions. This simple fact shows why a balanced diet is so important.

As a guide to discovering which foods are supplying what amounts of essential nutrients in the average American diet, a set of tables has been included at the end of this chapter. The tables, from the NHANES II (Second National Health and Nutrition Examination Survey), are extremely illuminating because they reveal individual nutrient supplies from foods by the quantities in which they are consumed rather than by the food's nutrient "quality."

CoQ Supplies from Animals

Beef muscle and heart are rich sources of CoQ_{10}. But not all of our food supplies are so abundant in CoQ_{10}, the form of coenzyme Q that is essential to humans. In Chapter 2 is a brief synopsis of some of the occurrences of coenzyme Q in nature. Here they are listed in detail.

Just about everything eaten by the human will contain various members of the coenzyme Q family, the ubiquinones. But only some of these ubiquinones may actually be CoQ_{10}. However, the internal biochemistry of the liver will utilize these other coenzyme Qs (most of them lower numbers on the Q scale—CoQ_9, CoQ_8, or CoQ_7 for example), taking them apart and splicing them together to form CoQ_{10}s, providing the body's ability to perform this task has not declined. The lack of the ability to perform this internal chemical conversion to CoQ_{10} is a crucial factor in why some people become deficient in CoQ_{10} as they grow older. This process is discussed in more detail in the section on CoQ supplements in this chapter.

As a guide to the importance of CoQ relative to the individual organs and tissues of the human body, the first table (Table I) will serve as an illustration. It shows which organs and tissues were first found to contain high concentrations of CoQ. The second table (Table II) lists different animals and the areas within their bodies that scientists intitially identified as containing CoQ_{10}.

*Note: these tables reflect preliminary scientific findings. Updated and more precise tables have since been developed and follow later in this chapter.

TABLE I

Naturally Occurring CoQ_{10} in Man

	Tissue
Man	Heart
	Liver
	Kidney
	Spleen
	Pancreas
	Skeletal muscle
	Blood
	Blood plasma
	Urine

In Table II it's easy to spot the potentially richer sources of direct CoQ_{10} in the average diet and also notice that many of these sources are edible animal parts that are often discarded as unpalatable in the regular diet.

TABLE II

Naturally Occurring CoQ_{10} in Animal Tissues

Animal	Tissue
Cow	Heart
	Liver
	Kidney
	Spleen
	Pancreas
	Skeletal muscle
	Milk fat
Pig	Liver
	Heart
	Spleen
	Pancreas
Sheep	Liver
	Heart
	Kidney
	Muscle
	Spleen
Rabbit	Liver
	Heart
Chicken	Heart
	Kidney
	Muscle
	Embryo (eggs)
Turkey	Heart
Cod	Liver
	Heart
Shrimp	(traces)

It becomes clear from this last table that beef (cow) is a prime source of CoQ, with the muscle, milk fat, heart, and liver all being good sources of the CoQ_{10} needed by man.

The muscle of chickens, sheep, and lamb all supply amounts

of CoQ_{10}. Eggs have been identified as containing significant amounts of CoQ. Because of their popularity in a great variety of individual dishes, and their place as an essential ingredient in many recipes, eggs must therefore figure as a prime nutritional source of CoQ.

While the codfish is a good source of CoQ_{10}, it was only found in high concentrations in the liver and heart, which are normally discarded before cooking. Shrimps, however, do contain CoQ_{10} throughout their bodies but only in "trace" amounts.

These preliminary tables illustrate that good sources of CoQ_{10} are available within the wide range of available animal products.

Plants Containing CoQ

Some higher plants and vegetable oils also supply CoQ_{10}. Many of them are included in regular dietary habits, and these cannot be overlooked as an important overall source of CoQ, even though the individual amounts they contain may be exceedingly small.

CoQ_{10} and the lower CoQs also occur in a myriad of molds, fungi, yeasts, and microorganisms, but their contribution to our intake of CoQ through diet is probably minute.

Table III lists some of the first identified plant and vegetable oil sources of CoQ.

TABLE III

Naturally Occurring CoQs in Vegetables and Oils

Plant	CoQ
Spinach	CoQ_{10}
Alfalfa	CoQ_{10}
Potato	CoQ_{10}
Sweet potato	CoQ_{10}
Soybean	CoQ_{10}
Wheat seeds	CoQ_{10}
Safflower leaf	CoQ_9

Oils	CoQ
Rice bran oil	CoQ_{10}
Soybean oil	CoQ_{10}
Cottonseed oil	CoQ_{10}
Corn oil	CoQ_9
Wheat germ oil	CoQ_9

Research into the availability of CoQ through dietary means is still very much in its infancy. This should be kept in mind when reviewing these tables. Because a specific food source is not included does not mean that it doesn't contain CoQ_{10} or the other CoQs. For example, lobsters do not appear; neither do many types of fish, fowl such as duck and hens, game meats such as venison, and scores of different vegetables. They may well contain significant amounts of CoQ, but science has not identified them yet.

Latest Research Reveals Specific Food Contents in Many Foods

The previous tables detailed the earliest indications of CoQ content in a variety of food products, but very latest research breakthroughs now reveal a wealth of new CoQ information and its specific content for many popular foods in the regular diet. From these new tables we can draw more specific guidelines for obtaining adequate CoQ directly through the diet.

This information, collated by Japanese nutrition researchers, is so new that it wasn't made available until almost mid-1986 to Western scientists, and it is being presented here for the first time to the general public.

Using the most up-to-date techniques of biochemical analysis, scientists from the Department of Food Chemistry and Nutrition, Osaka City Institute of Public Health and Environmental Sciences, and the Department of Biochemistry at Osaka City University Medical School were able to identify the exact CoQ contents of many foods as diverse as cereals, legumes, nuts, vegetables, fish, and meat and dairy products. These breakthroughs were made possible by utilizing high-performance liquid chromatography, a very precise method of chemical analysis that can be adapted to recognizing specific nutrient combinations in foods.

The authors are indebted to Dr. M. Kamei and his team of researchers for supplying the following comprehensive tables, published in the *International Journal for Vitamin and Nutrition Research* (1986) under the title "The Distribution and Content of Ubiquinone in Foods." As all the foods contained in the tables are listed, one or two may be unknown to the Western dining table. But these unfamiliar exceptions have been included because of their availability at the speciality or gourmet counters in some food markets, or at stores specializing in ethnic, especially oriental, foodstuffs.

This important research, to quantify precisely ubiquinone content in our favorite foods, covers only the most important Q (for humans), Coenzyme Q_{10} and its nearest chemical "brother," Coenzyme Q_9. Not all foods and food categories have been analyzed in this initial research (most notably fruits and shellfish), but it is anticipated that ongoing studies by Japanese researchers soon will provide more eagerly awaited answers.

For the sake of simplicity, the CoQ contents are listed in milligrams per gram of food product. One thousand mg equal 1 gram. To make this equation even easier to understand, 100 grams of weight are equivalent to 3½ ounces (3.5 oz), or a little less than a quarter of a pound.

Take the example of the content of CoQ_{10} in beef. Beef is listed as containing .031 mg of CoQ_{10} for each gram of meat. Therefore, if we multiply .031 by 100, we obtain the CoQ content of 3.5 oz of beef—which is 3.1 mg, or approximately 14 mg per pound of beef. To obtain a quick estimation of how much CoQ is contained in each 3.5-oz portion of the individually listed food, just move the decimal point two spaces to the right. For example, wheat germ, a highly significant source of CoQ (listed at .103 mg per gram), would contain 10.3 mg of CoQ_{10} per 3.5-oz serving; broccoli (listed at .0086 mg per gram) would yield .86 mg per 3.5-oz serving; while potatoes (listed at .001 gram per mg) would supply only .10 mg per 3.5-oz serving, or over 2 lbs of potatoes would be needed to provide just 1 mg of CoQ.

NOTE: It is well worth remembering that therapeutic dosages of pure, pharmaceutically produced CoQ_{10} range between 30 and 60 mg and up to 100 mg per day. Quality of CoQ content in individual food products may be significantly reduced by length of storage, processing, and methods of cooking.

Each of the tables is followed by a brief commentary.

TABLE IV
CoQ Content in Cereals

Food	Mg per Gm Dry Wt.	
	Q_9	Q_{10}
Rice		
Brown rice	.0048	—
Well-milled rice	.0026	—
Rice bran	.031	.0054
Wheat		
Whole grain	.0067	—
Wheat flour	.0015	—
Wheat germ	.103	.0035
Corn		
Whole grain	.025	—
Raw sweet	.039	—
Other cereals		
Barley (whole)	.011	—
Buckwheat (whole)	.021	.0013
Job's tears	.013	.0007
Oats (whole)	.013	—
Millet (whole)	.015	.0015

From these results it would appear that the "all-American" breakfast of cereals could supply surprisingly significant levels of CoQ, making it a potentially important meal of the day that shouldn't be missed.

Rice bran and especially wheat germ contain high quantities of Q_9 and smaller, but significant, amounts of Q_{10}. It is also apparent that the milling and refining process significantly reduces CoQ content, which indicates that its highest concentration is in the shells of the cereals. Corn, because it is very much a staple of the American diet, may prove to be an important supplier of coenzyme Q (see the entry for corn oil in Table X, "CoQ Content in Oils and Fats").

Breakfast cereals come in many varieties, including those made from rice brans and wheats, but it is clear that introducing additional wheat germ at breakfast can greatly increase potential CoQ benefits. Whole grain breads, or those containing wheat germ, also would yield high CoQ contents.

TABLE V

CoQ Content in Beans

Food	Mg per Gm Dry Wt.	
	Q_9	Q_{10}
Soybeans		
Whole, dry	—	.0021
Boiled	—	.0029
Green (raw)	—	.0058
Natto (fermented)	—	.0021
Kinako (roasted and ground)	.003	.0031
Azuki beans		
Whole, dry	.001	.0022

Soybean is now widely used, especially in meat replacement products. Soybean and soybean-based products, like tofu, are used in oriental cooking and are available at supermarkets and speciality stores.

The researchers make an important point that the processes of boiling, fermentation, and heat treatment do not appear to affect the effusion and destruction of CoQ in soybeans (see the entry for soybean oil in Table X). Other beans, more common to the traditional American diet, may contain similar amounts of CoQ.

TABLE VI

CoQ Content in Nuts and Seeds

Food	Mg per Gm Dry Wt.	
	Q_9	Q_{10}
Sweet almond (roasted)	.0063	.014
Pistachio (roasted)	—	.020
Peanuts (roasted)	—	.027
Hazelnuts (roasted)	—	.017
Walnuts (raw)	—	.019
Chestnuts (raw)	.0006	.014
Sesame seeds (roasted)	—	.023

Of all the nuts listed, peanuts rate the highest in levels of CoQ_{10}. This leads to the assumption that peanut butter may be a previously overlooked valuable source of CoQ in the American diet.

TABLE VII

CoQ Content in Vegetables

Food	Mg per Gm Wet Wt.	
	Q_9	Q_{10}
Cabbage	—	.0016
Broccoli	.0003	.0086
Rapeflower	—	.0074
Cauliflower	—	.0014
Chinese cabbage	—	.0010
Eggplant	—	.0021
Sweet pepper	.0002	.0033
Potato	—	.0010
Garlic	.0001	.0027
Onion	—	.0010
Leek	—	—
Sweet potato	—	.0036
Spinach	—	.010
Carrot	—	.0022
Perilla leaf (oriental mints)	—	.010
Lettuce	.0014	—
Edible burdock	.0036	—
Pumpkin	.0022	—
Cucumber	.0013	—
Basella	.0045	—

Spinach, long touted for its superior nutritional content, does it again—this time with its highly significant content of CoQ_{10}. Broccoli also is a good supply source of CoQ.

The researchers pointed out that most of the popular vegetables contain CoQ_{10} rather than CoQ_9.

TABLE VIII

CoQ Content in Fish

Food	Mg per Gm Wet Wt.		Mg per Gm Dry Wt.	
	Q_9	Q_{10}	Q_9	Q_{10}
Mackerel	—	.043	—	.104
Sardine	—	.064	—	.226
Horse mackerel	—	.020	—	.096
Yellowtail	.0003	.020	.0008	.023
Flatfish	—	.0055	—	.024
Eel	—	.011	—	.029
Cattlefish	.0006	.023	.029	.115

Both wet and dry weights have been included in this table, as some fish products are purchased dried and then reconstituted during preparation or the cooking process.

Mackerel and sardines contain the largest amounts of natural CoQ_{10} yet recognized in the food chain. And when these fish are dried, the concentration of CoQ increases dramatically in ratio to weight as the water content is reduced. As these are "oily" fish, it is fair to theorize that the content of CoQ is highest in oil-bearing tissues.

Fish in the native American diet that are recognized for their high oil content (such as salmon or cod) may be found to exhibit equally high volumes of CoQ_{10}.

TABLE IX
CoQ Content in Meats, Eggs, and Dairy Products

Food	Mg per Gm Wet Wt.	
	Q_9	Q_{10}
Meats		
Pork	—	.024 to .041
Chicken	—	.021
Beef	—	.031
Egg		
Chicken egg	—	.0037
Dairy products		
Butter	—	.0071
Cheese	—	.0021
Cow milk	.0002	.0004

Overall beef is the meat with the highest consistent content of CoQ. In some instances, pork supplies even higher amounts of CoQ and this may be directly related to the fluctuating concentration of CoQ in pork fatty tissue.

Because of their relatively high weight compared to volume, eggs may appear deceptively low in CoQ. But eggs are, in fact, good sources of CoQ_{10}.

Dairy products contain comparatively small amounts of CoQ among livestock products.

TABLE X
CoQ Content in Oils and Fats

Food	Mg per Gm Wet Wt.	
	Q_9	Q_{10}
Corn oil	.186	.013
Cottonseed oil	.059	.017
Safflower oil	.025	.0040
Sunflower oil	.021	.0042
Soybean oil	.008	.092
Sesame oil	—	.032
Rapeseed oil	.0021	.073
Olive oil	.0065	.0041
Rice bran oil	.0040	—
Coconut oil	—	—
Lard	—	.0010

When used as cooking oils or for deep frying, corn oil, soybean oil, rapeseed oil and sesame oil may impart significant amounts of CoQ into the diet, although it is uncertain how much a long-term heating process will affect overall CoQ content because of the result of the oxidation process at constant high temperatures. Quick stir-frying with these oils may help to preserve CoQ content. Olive oil showed little CoQ content.

Traces of CoQ were not detectable in coconut oil, which is commonly used in margarine products.

RDAs—Recommended Daily Allowances

More importantly, the RDAs (Recommended Daily Allowance) for CoQ_{10} have not yet been established. We can only speculate now as to the exact quantities of CoQ_{10} necessary for optimal health. But CoQ is no exception; for example, RDAs still are to be established for other essential nutritional factors, including choline, inositol, para-aminobenzoic acid (PABA), chromium, manganese, selenium, chloride, molybdenum, and others.

The nutritional application of CoQ_{10} is less than a decade old, and it will take many more years for researchers to analyze every food source for CoQ content. At the moment scientists have concentrated on obvious ones, but this does not mean that there won't be any future surprises. Foods such as lobster, or the various members of the shellfish family, that have not yet been quantified for their CoQ_{10} content may prove to be bountiful sources.

At present the best advice to follow for ensuring adequate supplies of CoQ_{10} in the diet is to eat well-balanced meals that include a variety of beef, chicken, pork, and egg dishes; fish, especially mackerel and sardines; cereals, especially the brans; nuts, such as peanuts and peanut butter: and also CoQ_{10}-rich vegetables such as broccoli and spinach.

The very latest nutritional information on the CoQ_{10} content of oils also indicates that valuable sources of the coenzyme may be obtained by utilizing oils such as soybean oil, rapeseed oil, and sesame oil in dishes, or with salads.

The Most Viable Alternative

An alternative method to supplying CoQ_{10} totally through nutrition is to take CoQ_{10} supplements as an adjunct to the regular diet. Because CoQ_{10} supplements come in specific quantities, it is therefore easy to judge the "bonus" amounts of the nutrient being taken each day.

It is clear from the previous tables that Coenzyme Q_{10} can be derived from nature through the food chain, and the abundance of the other Qs act as a "back-up" source for CoQ_{10} when an individual is not getting sufficient amounts of the "human" CoQ.

But that leads to the problem of being able to make the necessary conversions of the other Qs into Q_{10}. Are adequate amounts of CoQ_{10} available through regular diet? No researcher knows for certain and this question will have to be answered by future scientific investigation.

One factor that points to an inability to obtain sufficient CoQ_{10} directly from the foods we eat is the inbuilt mechanism for converting the other Qs into CoQ_{10}. It could be said that if the human didn't need the other Qs, it wouldn't have developed the sophisticated chemistry to convert them into Q_{10}. Because it is now known that everybody's ability to make these conversions varies with age—with the possibility of a significant decline in advanced age—this poses a distinct quandary.

The problem is twofold: how to recognize at what age an individual may begin to lose the ability to produce CoQ, and at what time in chronological aging it may cease altogether. Because individuals vary, it is not possible to devise a predetermined scale of age related to ability to produce internal CoQ_{10}. Furthermore, the effect of diseases or drugs on natural CoQ_{10} levels within the human body has not yet been investigated fully, although a simple personal blood test may one day supply accurate answers.

Until a blood test, what can be done to protect against deficiencies of CoQ? There is a solution, and that is to take supplemental CoQ.

All the studies throughout this book have utilized supplemental CoQ to correct deficiency states, mostly as simple as adding supplements to the regular diet, and on a few occasions by injection.

Oral CoQ supplements have the advantage that they are

portable, can be taken together with meals, and will digest naturally along with other foods. Injected supplements have the advantage of being administered directly into the bloodstream's transportation mechanism with the potential of being absorbed faster where CoQ may be needed the most.

CoQ supplements are now available over-the-counter (OTC) in many health food stores and in the vitamin sections of pharmacies and supermarkets. But it must be stressed that no health benefits can be claimed for CoQ supplements by the manufacturers, suppliers, or, for that matter, by the authors of this book. This is because CoQ has not been placed by the FDA in any drug classification, as yet. No therapeutic benefits can be claimed for CoQ until the FDA has reviewed and accepted exhaustive studies that have proved lack of toxicity and beneficial applications. The FDA can then authorize its sale as a "therapeutic." In the case of CoQ it would then also be available as a prescription drug.

Classification as a prescription drug would offer many advantages to CoQ therapy. Among them are the following:

• It would bring CoQ to the attention of medical practitioners who would have the benefit of therapeutic guidelines.

• It would identify specifically the state of ill health or disease for which a particular CoQ preparation had been targeted.

• Dosages would be defined for various therapeutic usages.

• The public would be clearly informed (either through the medical profession or pharmaceutical literature accompanying the product) what health benefits to expect.

Nevertheless, CoQ is available and is marketed as a dietary supplement without any health claims, and therefore without the necessity for FDA clearance. However, nobody should take CoQ as medication for an already diagnosed medical problem. *You must consult your physician* if you intend to take this course of action. *It is dangerous to self-medicate.*

If the reader wants to embark on a course of CoQ supplementation, it is urged that you talk with your physician first and the authors strongly suggest that you take this book along with you as an informational and reference guide for your physician.

Supplies

The average bottle of one hundred 10 mg capsules of CoQ_{10} (a 3 month supply if ingested at 10 mg a day) will retail at between $16 and $18. CoQ in fifty capsule units of 10 mg retails for approximately $9. CoQ_{10} supplies into the United States have so far been limited, but as competition in the CoQ_{10} marketplace increases to meet demand the retail price is expected to be eventually forced down.

At present the authors know of only one supplier in the United States importing pure pharmaceutical CoQ_{10} directly from Japan and encapsulating in this country. This company is TwinLabs of Ronkonkoma, Long Island, New York. Since CoQ is used in Japan mainly as a prescription drug, production from Japanese chemical and pharmaceutical companies is under strict control for purity and effectiveness.

How Much CoQ

It is not ethical for the authors to prescribe any dosages of CoQ_{10} on a therapeutic basis. A physician may prescribe CoQ_{10}, but, like any other drug, he will want to evaluate the severity of the disease or medical problem, the use of other drugs in combination, and general health status before making any recommendation. But a review of the literature in this book suggests that a regular daily maintenance dosage of CoQ_{10} ranges from 10 to 30 mg, while more serious states of CoQ_{10} deficiency have been shown to respond well to dosages of up to and over 100 mg a day.

However, it is worth remembering at this point that no toxicity tests of CoQ_{10} have shown any adverse side effects even at continual dosages many times the therapeutic levels used in clinical studies.

Capsules Versus Tablets

In early studies by Japanese biochemists from the Eisai Pharmaceutical Company it was found that gelatin capsules provided the most efficient, optimal form for CoQ_{10} release. Tablet forms of CoQ_{10} were discarded during early clinical research by Japanese manufacturers because many of the combinations were found to be ineffective as release agents for CoQ_{10}. Tablets require binders which may slow down the absorption process, or, as in some cases, inhibit it altogether so that the bound CoQ_{10} pass through the alimentary canal without being absorbed at all. Capsules are therefore the preferred vehicle for CoQ_{10} at the present time.

Buyer Beware!

As the demand for CoQ_{10} increases, it can be expected that a rash of CoQ_{10} products will enter the market. And not all of these will be offering the purest of CoQ_{10}.

Many products may advertise themselves as CoQ_{10}, but contain only minute amounts of the nutrient with fillers like cornmeal, soybean meal, yeast, wheatmeal, milk or egg derivatives, together with sugars, flavors, and coloring. They might look like CoQ_{10}, but their CoQ_{10} content may be so minuscule as to be totally ineffective. Beware of products that may advertise themselves with names that sound like Coenzyme Q_{10}. Examples might be C-10, Co_{10}, Q, coenzyme Q (which could imply any of the other CoQ's), enzyme Q, Q Formula, and any other variety of combinations.

A guideline for recognizing pure CoQ_{10} is that its natural color is a bright yellow, bordering on orange. It has little appreciable taste in its powdered state.

Available CoQ Products

The following is a list of available CoQ products. Evaluations are based on information supplied by individual distributors.

Brand name: Maxilife CoQ_{10} Formula

Producer: Twin Laboratories, Inc.
2120 Smithtown Ave.
Ronkonkoma, N.Y. 11779

Contents: Each capsule contains 10 mg pure Coenzyme Q_{10}, in a formula that includes vitamins E, C, and the Bs, together with selenium, zinc, and other antioxidants.

Recommended dose: 2 capsules per day, or as recommended by a physician.

Availability: 6,000 health food stores nationwide.

Comment: The most comprehensive CoQ antiaging and antioxidant formula on the market.

Brand name: CoQ$_{10}$

Producer: Twin Laboratories, Inc.
         2120 Smithtown Avenue
         Ronkonkoma, N.Y. 11779

Contents: Each capsule contains 10 mg pure Coenzyme Q$_{10}$.

Recommended dose: 1 to 3 capsules per day as a dietary supplement.

Availability: 6,000 health food stores nationwide.

Comment: Pharmaceutically pure CoQ$_{10}$ which in recommended dosages will supply sufficient daily levels of supplemental CoQ$_{10}$.

Brand name: CoQ-Plus Aging Formula

Supplier: Dajean Gerontological Labs
         P.O. Box 314
         Lake Grove, N.Y. 11755

Contents: Each capsule contains 10 mg pure Coenzyme Q$_{10}$ in a vitamin rich antioxidant formula.

Recommended dose: 2 capsules a day, or as directed by a physician.

Availability: Mail order only. CoQ information booklet also available on request.

Comment: A superior formula of antiaging and antioxidant nutrients containing accepted therapeutic levels of CoQ.

Brand name: Co-Q-Mulsion

Supplier: Biotics Research Corporation*
         5731 Savoy Lane
         Houston, Texas 77036
         Tel: (713) 789-9020

*Note: Biotics Research Corporation has variously described its source of CoQ as "a specially grown biologically active vegetable culture," and "from young bovine heart tissue." The supplier claims that the reason for small CoQ content in its products is because the CoQ source provides for higher biological activity, but no technical information is provided to justify the claim. This fact may cause confusion when attempting to assess actual CoQ efficacy.

Contents: Each 10 drops supply 50 mcg of coenzyme Q and 10 IU of vitamin E.

Recommended dose: 10 to 30 drops each day.

Availability: Mail order or through regional suppliers.

Comment: An emulsified version of CoQ. Minute content of CoQ suggests that at least 200 times the supplier's recommended dosage would be necessary before the established therapeutic dose of 10 mg is reached. Supplier describes active ingredient as coenzyme Q.

Brand name: Coenzyme Q_{10} Forte

Supplier: Biotics Research Corporation*
    5731 Savoy Lane
    Houston, Texas 77036
    Tel: (713) 789-9020

Content: Each tablet contains 1 mg of coenzyme Q, 30 mcg of superoxide dismutase, and 30 mcg catalase.

Recommended dose: 1 to 3 tablets each day.

Availability: Mail order or through regional suppliers.

Comment: Low levels of CoQ. Single dose would have to be increased tenfold to supply 10 mg of CoQ, but this would also mean that the other ingredients (superoxide dismutase and catalase) are also increased to possibly unwanted levels. Active ingredient described by supplier as Coenzyme Q_{10}.

Brand name: Bio-Multi Plus

Supplier: Biotics Research Corporation*
    5731 Savoy Lane
    Houston, Texas 77036
    Tel: (713) 789-9020

---

*Note: Biotics Research Corporation has variously described its source of CoQ as "a specially grown biologically active vegetable culture," and "from young bovine heart tissue." The supplier claims that the reason for small CoQ content in its products is because the CoQ source provides for higher biological activity, but no technical information is provided to justify the claim. This fact may cause confusion when attempting to assess actual CoQ efficacy.

Content: 3 tablets contain a multivitamin and mineral combination that includes 25 mcg of coenzyme Q.

Recommended dose: 3 tablets per day.

Availability: Mail order or through regional suppliers.

Comment: Extremely low dosages of CoQ. 120 tablets would have to be consumed before 1 mg of CoQ would be reached, but this might supply undesirably high levels of other nutrients.

Brand name: Coenzyme Q$_{10}$

Supplier: Cardiovascular Research, Ltd.
        1061-B Shary Circle
        Concorde, Calif. 94518
        Tel: (415) 827-2636

Content: Each capsule contains 10 mg of pure, reduced Coenzyme Q$_{10}$.

Recommended dose: One capsule daily, or as directed by a physician.

Availability: Mail order, health food stores and pharmacies.

Comment: The supplier warns that "due to its low melting point, Co-enzyme Q$_{10}$ should be kept away from heat or light." The melting point of pure Coenzyme Q$_{10}$ is 49 degrees centigrade, or approximately 115 degrees Fahrenheit.

Brand name: Free Radical Quenchers

Supplier: Cardiovascular Research Ltd.
        1061-B Shary Circle
        Concord, Calif. 94518
        Tel: (415) 827-2636

Content: Each capsule contains a mixture of antioxidant nutrients including 500 mcg of "Ubiquinone."

Recommended dose: One capsule daily, or as directed by a physician.

Availability: Mail order, health food stores and pharmacies.

Comment: Low content of CoQ. 2 capsules would supply only 1 mg of CoQ.

Nutrients Supplied in the Average American Diet

Listed in this section is each of the top 50 foods that supply vitamins A, B_1 (thiamine), B_2 (riboflavin), B_3 (niacin), and C, and minerals, iron, phosphorus, calcium, sodium, and potassium. It is important to note that these are the foods that supply most of these nutrients by virtue of the amounts of these foods that are eaten—they do not indicate that the foods are individually the richest sources of the nutrient.

For example, French fries, potatoes, greens, and tomatoes are valuable suppliers of vitamin C because of the large amounts of these foods that are consumed. They might generally be overlooked as valuable dietary sources of C because of their small content of the vitamin—but overall they rank high as important providers.

The following tables were compiled from the NHANES II study by Dr. Gladys Block, a member of the Surveillance and Operations Research Branch of the Division of Cancer Prevention and Control at the National Cancer Institute, and offer for the first time a fascinating view of what foods are actually supplying which nutrients in the American diet.

Remember, these tables apply to the average way Americans eat. They represent a sampling that corresponds to the diets of 132 million Americans. The figures in parentheses for the first ten foods in each group show the average percentage of the nutrient supplied each day by that particular food source. The foods without percentages specified follow in descending order of importance.

Vitamin A
Top ten: liver (12.53); carrots (8.43); eggs (6.04); tomatoes, tomato juice (4.65); vegetable, tomato, minestrone soups (4.04); whole milk, whole milk beverages (3.82); greens (mustard,

turnip, collards) (3.44); cantaloupe (3.20); margarine (3.04); cold cereals, excluding bran or superfortified types (3.01).

Next forty (in descending order of importance): spinach; cheeses, excluding cottage cheese; green salad; spaghetti with tomato sauce; orange juice; 2% milk (meaning 2% milk fat); sweet potatoes; beef stew, pot pie; mixed vegetables; butter; superfortified cold cereals; skim milk, buttermilk; ice cream, frozen desserts; peaches; broccoli; bran and granola cereals; liverwurst; soups other than vegetable, tomato; corn; doughnuts, cookies, cake; pumpkin pie; fortified fruit drinks; green beans; fortified orange juice substitutes; watermelon; chicken or turkey, excluding fried; pizza; catsup, other products with tomatoes; mixed dishes with cheese; winter squash; peas; potatoes, excluding fried; oranges, tangerines; grapefruits, grapefruit juice; hamburgers, cheeseburgers, meat loaf; cornbread, grits, tortillas; apricots; mixed dishes with chicken; bananas; breakfast bars and drinks.

Vitamin B_1 (thiamine)

White bread, rolls, crackers (17.81); pork, including chops, roasts (8.87); hot dogs, ham, lunch meats (5.37); cold cereals, excluding bran or superfortified types (4.48); orange juice (3.86); doughnuts, cookies, cake (3.45); whole milk, whole milk beverages (3.43); whole wheat, rye, other dark breads (2.90); hamburgers, cheeseburgers, meat loaf (2.71); breakfast bars and drinks (2.26).

French fries, fried potatoes; pinto, navy, other dried beans; potatoes, excluding fried; eggs; spaghetti with tomato sauce; bran and granola cereals; superfortified cold cereals; beef steaks, roasts; 2% milk; tomatoes, tomato juice; skim milk, buttermilk; sausage; green salad; pizza; cornbread, grits, tortillas; bacon; salty snacks; rice; pies, excluding pumpkin; cooked cereals; oranges, tangerines; peanuts, peanut butter; corn; ice cream, frozen desserts; grapefruit, grapefruit juice; chicken or turkey, excluding fried; beef stew, pot pie; soups, excluding vegetable, tomato; peas; fried fish; cheeses, excluding cottage; mixed dishes with cheese; noodles, macaroni; pancakes, waffles, French toast; fried chicken; apples, applesauce; bananas; candy (chocolate); liver; vegetable, tomato, minestrone soups.

Vitamin B₂ (riboflavin)

Whole milk, whole milk beverages (13.38); white bread, rolls, crackers, (8.57); 2% milk (6.47); hamburgers, cheeseburgers, meat loaf (4.44); eggs (4.28); beef steaks, roasts (4.17); skim milk, buttermilk (4.12); liver (3.69); cheeses, excluding cottage (3.51); cold cereals, excluding bran or superfortified types (3.38).

Some alcoholic beverages; doughnuts, cookies, cake; hot dogs, ham, lunch meats; ice cream, frozen desserts; pork, including chops, roasts; breakfast bars and drinks; superfortified cold cereals; spaghetti with tomato sauce; bran and granola cereals; whole wheat, rye, other dark breads; fried chicken; green salad; chicken or turkey, excluding fried; fortified fruit drinks; coffee, tea; potatoes, excluding fried; cornbread, grits, tortillas; pizza; tomatoes, tomato juice; mixed dishes with cheese; pies, excluding pumpkin; soups other than vegetable, tomato; yogurt; pinto, navy, other dried beans; cottage cheese; chili; French fries, fried potatoes; pancakes, waffles, French toast; corn; beef stew, pot pie; fried fish; sausage; liverwurst; orange juice; candy (chocolate); bacon; cream, half-and-half; tuna, tuna salad, tuna casserole; puddings; fish, broiled, baked, canned.

Vitamin B₃ (niacin)

White bread, rolls, crackers (9.51); beef steaks, roasts (8.49); coffee, tea (7.93); hamburgers, cheeseburgers, meat loaf (7.58); alcoholic beverages, especially beer (5.00); chicken or turkey, excluding fried (4.56); cold cereals, excluding bran or superfortified types (3.82); pork, including chops, roasts (3.73); fried chicken (3.66); hot dogs, ham, lunch meats (3.33).

French fries, fried potatoes; peanuts, peanut butter; doughnuts, cookies, cake; potatoes, excluding fried; tuna, tuna salad, tuna casseroles; spaghetti with tomato sauce; whole wheat, rye, other dark breads; bran and granola cereals; superfortified cold cereals; liver; cheeses, excluding cottage; beef stew, pot pie; orange juice; tomatoes, tomato juice; breakfast bars and drinks; fried fish; fish, broiled, baked, canned; whole milk, whole milk beverages; pizza; salty snacks; chili; skim milk, buttermilk; corn; rice; bacon; pinto, navy, other dried beans; veal, lamb; soups other than vegetable, tomato; cornbread, grits, tortillas; green salads; sausage; vegetable, tomato, minestrone soups; pies, excluding pumpkin; mixed dishes with chicken; shellfish; mixed dishes with beef; candy (chocolate); bananas; 2% milk; peaches.

Vitamin C

Orange juice (26.54); grapefruit, grapefruit juice (7.20); tomatoes, tomato juice (6.12); fortified fruit drinks (5.85); oranges, tangerines (4.90); potatoes, excluding fried (4.20); French fries, fried potatoes (4.08); green salads (3.49); other fruit juices (2.81); broccoli (1.98).

Coleslaw, cabbage; spaghetti with tomato sauce; fortified orange juice substitutes; cold cereals, excluding bran or superfortified types; hot dogs, ham, lunch meats; cantaloupe; whole milk, whole milk beverages; greens (mustard, turnips, collards); strawberries; superfortified cold cereals; bananas; beef stew, pot pie; corn; 2% milk; lemons, lemon juice; spinach; apples, apple sauce; liver; green beans; bacon; peas; green peppers; pinto, navy, other dried beans; pizza; vegetable, tomato, minestrone soups; salty snacks; peaches; cauliflower; watermelon; bran, and granola cereals; carrots; catsup, other products with tomatoes; mixed vegetables; chili peppers, hot chili sauce; brussels sprouts; sweet potatoes; skim milk, buttermilk; jellies, jams, honey; gelatin dessert; fruit cocktail, fruit salad.

Iron

White bread, rolls, crackers (11.43); beef steaks, roasts (9.04); hamburgers, cheeseburgers, meat loaf (6.90); eggs (4.16); coffee, tea (4.05); pork, including chops, roasts (3.59); doughnuts, cookies, cake (3.34); hot dogs, ham, lunch meats (3.26); cold cereals, excluding bran or superfortified types (3.11); pinto, navy, other dried beans (2.66).

Spaghetti with tomato sauce; French fries, fried potatoes; whole wheat, rye, other dark breads; superfortified cold cereals; bran and granola cereals; green salad; liver; chili; potatoes, excluding fried; chicken or turkey, excluding fried; cooked cereals; tomatoes, tomato juice; fried chicken; beef stew, pot pie; cornbread, grits, tortillas; pizza; cheeses, excluding cottage; soups other than vegetable, tomato; salty snacks; pies, excluding pumpkin; rice; fried fish; shellfish; tuna, tuna salad, tuna casserole; vegetable, tomato, minestone soups; green beans; grapefruit, grapefruit juice; orange juice; peas; corn; peanuts, peanut butter; bananas; 2% milk; breakfast bars and drinks; sausage; apples, applesauce; mixed dishes with beef; fish, broiled, baked, canned; mixed dishes with cheese; prunes.

Phosphorus

Whole milk, whole milk beverages (10.46); cheeses, excluding cottage (6.04); white bread, rolls, crackers (5.69); beef steaks, roasts (5.58); 2% milk (5.00); hamburgers, cheeseburgers, meat loaf (4.68); eggs (4.36); alcoholic beverages (4.15); skim milk, buttermilk (3.38); doughnuts, cookies, cake (2.94).

Pork, including chops, roast; hot dogs, ham, lunch meats; whole wheat, rye, other dark breads; chicken or turkey, excluding fried; pinto, navy, other dried beans; coffee, tea; spaghetti with tomato sauce; ice cream, frozen desserts; French fries, fried potatoes; fried chicken; potatoes, excluding fried; fried fish; bran, and granola cereals; chili; cornbread, grits, tortillas; peanuts, peanut butter; fish, broiled, baked, canned; regular soft drinks; orange juice; cold cereals, excluding bran or superfortified types; pizza; salty snacks; tuna, tuna salad, tuna casserole; beef stew, pot pie; soups other than vegetable, tomato; corn; mixed dishes with cheese; green salad; cottage cheese; tomatoes, tomato juice; liver; bacon; candy (chocolate); shellfish; cooked cereals; pancakes, waffles, French toast; rice; yogurt; fortified fruit drinks; sausage.

Calcium

Whole milk, whole milk beverages (21.97); cheeses, excluding cottage cheese (12.01); 2% milk (10.55); white bread, rolls, crackers (8.39); skim milk, buttermilk (6.88); ice cream, frozen desserts (3.34); eggs (2.38); doughnuts, cookies, cake (1.91); whole wheat, rye, other dark breads (1.62); spaghetti with tomato sauce (1.47).

Coffee, tea; some alcoholic beverages; cornbread, grits, tortillas; hamburgers, cheeseburgers, meat loaf; mixed dishes with cheese; pizza; pinto, navy, other dried beans; green salad; yogurt; potatoes, excluding fried; soups other than vegetable, tomato; orange juice; candy (chocolate); pancakes, waffles, French toast; cream, half-and-half; greens; puddings; beef steaks, roasts; oranges, tangerines; tomatoes, tomato juice; cottage cheese; chili; coleslaw, cabbage; green beans; fish, broiled, baked, canned; breakfast bars and drinks; shellfish; grapefruit, grapefruit juice; pies, excluding pumpkin; fortified fruit drinks; salty snacks; French fries, fried potatoes; cooked cereals; hot dogs, ham, lunch meats; vegetable, tomato, minestrone soups; spinach; fried fish; cold cereals, excluding bran or superfortified types; peanuts, peanut butter; rice.

Sodium

White bread, rolls, crackers (12.09); hot dogs, ham, lunch meats (9.76); cheeses, excluding cottage (5.37); soups other than vegetable, tomato (4.04); spaghetti with tomato sauce (3.61); doughnuts, cookies, cake (3.57); potatoes, excluding fried (3.28); vegetable, tomato, minestrone soups (2.64); eggs (2.56); whole milk, whole milk beverages (2.47).

Whole wheat, rye, other dark breads; chili; hamburgers, cheeseburgers, meat loaf; mayonnaise, salad dressings; French fries, fried potatoes; salty snacks; margarine; cornbread, grits, tortillas; pizza; rice; pork, including chops, roast; pinto, navy, other dried beans; cold cereals, excluding bran or superfortified types; 2% milk; bacon; beef steaks, roasts; tuna, tuna salad, tuna casserole; mixed dishes with cheese; pies, excluding pumpkin; catsup, other products with tomatoes; gravy, other meat sauces; sausage; corn; coleslaw, cabbage; butter; skim milk, buttermilk; fish, broiled, baked, canned; mixed dishes with beef; beef stew, pot pie; mixed dishes with chicken; cooked cereals; cottage cheese; pancakes, waffles, French toast; green beans; chicken or turkey, excluding fried; tomatoes, tomato juice; bran and granola cereals; ice cream, frozen desserts; fried fish; peanuts, peanut butter.

Potassium

Coffee, tea (8.63); whole milk, whole milk beverages (8.18); French fries, fried potatoes (5.67); orange juice (4.53); potatoes, excluding fried (4.29); 2% milk (3.92); beef steaks, roasts (3.90); hamburgers, cheeseburgers, meat loaf (3.17); tomatoes, tomato juice (2.72); white bread, rolls, crackers (2.67).

Skim milk, buttermilk; green salad; spaghetti with tomato sauce; some alcoholic beverages; pinto, navy, other dried beans; hot dogs, ham, lunch meats; pork, including chops, roast; chicken or turkey, excluding fried; eggs; ice cream, frozen desserts; doughnuts, cookies, cake; salty snacks; bananas; grapefruit, grapefruit juice; beef stew, pot pie; fried chicken; whole wheat, rye, other dark breads; chili, fried fish; cheeses, excluding cottage; peanuts, peanut butter; oranges, tangerines; bran and granola cereals; vegetable, tomato, minestrone soups; apples, applesauce; soups other than vegetable, tomato; fish, broiled, baked, canned; corn; coleslaw, cabbage; cantaloupe; other fruit juices; peaches; tuna, tuna salad, tuna casserole; carrots, peas and carrots; cold cereals, excluding bran or superfortified types; candy (chocolate); pizza; cornbread, grits, tortillas; pies, excluding pumpkin; yogurt.

Vitamins D and E were not included in the NHANES II survey of favorite American foods for two reasons: most vitamin D comes from sunlight or through vitamin D fortified milk, vitamin E mainly from vegetables and seed oils—and it is generally accepted that the average American diet supplies more than enough of these needs.

But it must be emphasized that the role of vitamin E (and boosting vitamin E intake by supplements) is being increasingly recognized as of prime importance for optimal immune system function. This is discussed in detail in the immune system chapter, Chapter 3.

CHAPTER 14

·

CoQ and Life Extension

"Probably no subject so deeply interests human
beings as that of the duration of life."
Raymond Pearl—*The Biology of Death*

The expectation of life is a haunting enigma to every single
person. And it is true to say that one will never know his own
true potential until that very last moment of ultimate individual finality. This is what makes life span such a curious
phenomenon.

Life has so many varieties of time span that no individual is
expected, or would even want to, accurately predict his own
demise to the hour, day, year, or even the decade. Yet there
are factors that control it, and one of those may be the
availability of CoQ at the cellular level.

The crux of all life extension is to prolong existence, but to
live longer in ill health or diseased states might be a futile
task. CoQ's potential shows the ability to not only lengthen
life, but to prolong the quality of that life.

The essence of old age is a cruel paradox. To grow old is to
be wise; to be youthful is to be foolish. To age is also to be
infirm and weak, while to be young is strength and agility.
There are two distinct viewpoints on aging; one is mental,
the other physical. If it were possible to combine the best of
both attributes, a sharper, more experienced mind in a healthier than expected body, it might indeed be something akin to
the legendary Fountain of Youth. It is from this perspective
that we should all approach the problem of aging; long life is
not necessarily advantageous if it is not accompanied by the
all important quality of good health.

Predictions from the National Institute on Aging show that
if current trends continue, we can expect large increases in

life expectancy at older ages. By the year 2000, there will be approximately 35.8 million people over 65, and life expectancy at birth will be 80.4 years. Possibly the most important prediction is that people who survive to age 65 can look forward to another 21.8 years of life!

There is probably no other area of biological inquiry that is underpinned by so many theories than gerontology, the science of aging. This is due in part to the lack of fundamental scientific data in the field. When we begin to experiment with human longevity, we surely cannot expect to see results for many years. Just as aging is a slow, and mostly unremitting process, so is the study of it.

That CoQ plays a crucial role in aging is beyond doubt. The same also applies to CoQ's role in the immune system. And there is a vital connection between the immune system and aging that cannot be ignored. Out of our many studies at the New England Institute one stands out when other researchers look to illustrate the life extension benefits of coenzyme Q. Its result was inspiring.

These experiments were briefly mentioned in Chapter 3 because of their important links with the immune system, and are discussed in detail in the next section.

Instant results cannot be expected in the study of human gerontology. With small animals as models, the whole story is much shorter on the time scale. It was with female white mice that a possible view of the Fountain of Youth was experienced.

Extending Life by Fifty Percent

It should first be explained that the study involved "old mice." The term means that these mice are already at such an advanced age that all their body functions are declining. Old mice have already lost their thymuses, show dramatic CoQ deficiency, and their immune systems have lost the capability to produce antibodies.

A mouse is considered to have reached "old" when it is approximately 16 to 18 months of age. In human terms this might be equivalent to being in one's sixties or seventies. It might make it easier to consider a week in the life of a mouse as roughly equivalent to 1 year in that of a human. A mouse living to 2 years would be like humans living well into their 90s.

For our study we took one hundred old mice, average age 16 to 18 months, and divided them into two groups of 50 each. Both groups were kept on optimally nutritious diets, and, in mouse terms, their life-styles and living conditions could be considered comfortable, or above average. Nothing had previously been done to extend their potential life spans beyond the expected norm.

At the start of the experiment, one group was selected as a control, and the remaining 50 mice were individually injected with CoQ each week. The CoQ was administered into the peritoneum in a harmless injectable emulsion. What soon became most apparent between the two groups was that the CoQ-treated mice did not develop the normally expected signs of advanced age. For example, their coats remained lustrous and healthy. They were bright-eyed and active, and showed none of the immobility problems associated with old age in mice.

The untreated mice lacked vigor and their fur grew sparse and patchy. They began to die at an expected rate. By week 16 of the experiment almost 30 percent of the control mice had succumbed to natural aging, while only 20 percent of the treated mice had died. From this point on the disparity between the two groups began to widen enormously.

By week 28 about 40 percent of the CoQ mice had died, compared to almost 70 percent of the control mice. At week 36 all members of the control group .were dead—yet almost 40 percent of the CoQ-treated mice were alive and active, and most of them displayed no observable signs of aging at a time when they should have been severely geriatric. The CoQ-treated mice continued their extraordinary odyssey of life. By week 56 (almost twice as long as they normally would be expected to survive beyond the start of the experiment) 10 percent were still thriving. As the study progressed toward its 80th week (remember, the last control mouse died at week 36), some 3 or 4 mice were still alive. The last CoQ-treated mouse finally died of "old age" at week 82—a life span which could be considered in human terms to be around 150 years!

The following table, Table I, shows the average survival times of the untreated and CoQ-treated mice.

TABLE I

Modification of Mean Survival Time in Old Mice by Coenzyme
Q_{10}

Treatment	Mean Survival Time after Treatment	
	Weeks	Percent
Control	20.0	100.0
LCoenzyme Q_{10}	31.2	156.0

And Chart A illustrates the survival times of the CoQ-treated mice compared to the controls. When these results were analyzed by computer they were found to be not just significant, but highly significant.

One of the most exciting facts about the CoQ treatment was that not only did it extend the average age expectancy of ordinary laboratory mice by at least half a lifetime, but the animals retained a more youthful appearance right up to the end of their lives.

In human terms these results could be interpreted as everybody having the potential to live to an average of 100 years instead of around 70, and some people could be expected to top 130 and even 150 years of age. Yet we must remember one important thing: no attempts were made in these experiments to counter any disease states that were not CoQ dependent and that may lead to death. Looking at that fact in a human situation, where disease states could be treated accordingly, the prospects of life extension could be even greater.

These experiments were repeated two more times to authenticate them with similar results. The preliminary CoQ and aging experiments were presented at the 4th International Congress of Immunology, in Paris, France, in 1980. The final detailed results were published in *Biochemical and Clinical Aspects of Coenzyme Q*, volume 3, in 1981.

Searching for the Secrets of Aging

You're only as young as your immune system. This thought-provoking statement is quoted by many researchers in the immune field. Scientists now attach a crucial importance to the link between the immune system and aging.

CHART A

Modification of Overall Age-Related Mortality in Old Mice by Coenzyme Q Treatment

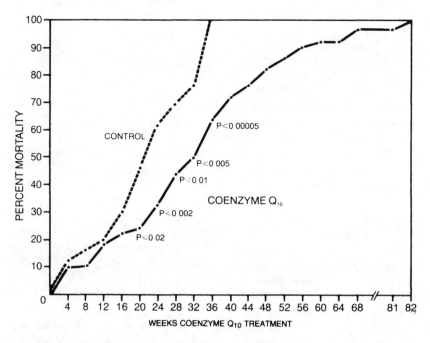

P = Significance Factor (i.e. P<0.02 is significant, P<0.00005 is extremely significant)

There is nothing so wonderful as having experienced a full and rewarding lifetime—to be in old age and still have good health. We marvel at the elderly who are in prime physical and mental shape. We use expressions like "He's still as sharp as a tack" or "She's as bright as a button" without really considering why this should be so.

It has become increasingly obvious that old people who survive life's complications into their 70s and 80s have had far fewer incidences of illness and disease states. And it becomes equally obvious that they must have had particularly strong immune systems to achieve this feat of stamina and endurance.

The surprise is always the centenarian who boasts of having enjoyed every minute of his life while smoking each day and imbibing modest quantities of alcohol. This is not the longevity stereotype expected.

The person with this type of life-style must surely have had something extraordinary going for him. It may now come as no surprise to discover that this individual suffered very little ill health throughout life, possibly because he was endowed with an immune system that could be considered superior in its efficiency.

As the human body progresses through the various stages of aging it is exposed to a large number of health pitfalls, which a weak or deficient immune system can have problems coping with. A demanding state of ill health—for example viral infections such as pneumonia, bronchitis, and even influenza—in early years, may leave immune "scars" that may not be too apparent until the immune system is called on to work overtime as the debilitating effects of aging become more overpowering.

Significant deficiencies are noticeable in the immune system as age passes. It is therefore in the organs of the immune system that we look for our first potential clues to the aging processes.

Immune Keys

In comparison to other studies in medicine, we are very ignorant of the aging process. This is due in part to the lack of fundamental scientific data in the field of gerontology. It is further complicated by the manifestation of the biological changes which, with time, affect all biological systems from the molecular level to the whole organism.

Although the age distribution of malignant disease encompasses the full range from the antenatal months to the ninth and tenth decades and beyond, neoplasia (the growth of tumor cells) is predominantly an occurrence of old age, just the time when the immune system is weakening.

There is now a growing body of evidence in favor of the concept that various "diseases of aging," including neoplasia, the immunodeficiency and autoimmunity, result from an involvement of major integrative systems. Those systems include, first, the immune and, second, the neurous and endocrine systems.

The association between immunodeficiency and increased cancer incidence is well established. When a patient is immunosuppressed, for example for organ transplantation, the cancer risk increases manyfold. Obviously, there is reason to believe that a decline in the immunological capability in the individual leads to an increased risk of cancer. We now know that such a decline occurs in all aging animals and humans.

The best known result of the decline of the immune system with aging is the impairment of the thymus function, which is under hormonal control, but which is also regulated by the brain. As a result of the important role of the thymus in spawning immune cells, the predominant immunological deficiency seen in the aging animal is a decline in the functions of the thymus-dependent T cells.

The T cells play a tremendously important role in the immune system. They have the dual role of marshaling the immune response (as helper cells) and also calling off the battle when no more immune fighters are needed (as suppressor cells). It's worth noting that the T cells are the same cells that fall victim to the disease of AIDS.

Some scientists have concluded that in mice the first event during aging is an increase in T cell suppressor function (possibly oversuppressing immune functions while they are still needed), followed by a decrease in T cell helper function. Because of the close connection between T and B cells, this finally results in a loss of B cell function.

All of this disrupts the immune system ratios of available T and B cells and the net result is a frighteningly weakened ability to generate maximal response to invading organisms.

In a joint study with Karl Folkers and his group at the University of Texas at Austin, we looked at one of the main immune organs, the thymus, in aged mice and compared it to young mice. A significant, sharp deficiency of CoQ activity was noticed in the thymus of the old mice.

The experiment involved 25, 10-week-old mice and a group of 75 old mice that were divided into three subgroups—the first being sacrificed at age 20 months, the second 2 months later (aged 22 months), and the third at 24 months. The thymuses were removed and weighed for the individual groups. It should be remembered that the thymus is the organ critical to the honing of T cells.

The ratio of thymus to body weight sharply decreased in the old mice. In fact, the 20-month-old mice had 57 percent the thymus weight of young mice, the 22-month-old, 45 percent, and the 24-month-old mice had only 23 percent of thymus weight compared to the youngsters. This clearly showed that the thymus was shrinking rapidly with the progression of old age.

It is known that exactly the same process happens in humans. After the age of 20 the thymus slowly shrinks and only traces of this vital organ are evident in elderly persons.

Furthermore, there was a marked acceleration of CoQ deficiency in the thymus of old animals. The sudden development in CoQ deficiency exactly mirrors the reduction of the thymus weight. At this dramatic deficiency level it is hard to expect that the thymus will perform any immunological function.

The following, Chart B, illustrates the obvious relationship between CoQ deficiency and thymus weight.

This established that aging results in a parallel deficiency of CoQ and shrinking of the thymus; the next step was to evaluate the capability of old mice to produce antibodies against a foreign antigen. Antibody response (immune protein fighting the disease) is one of the major and basic functions of the defense system.

In our experiments we took two groups of mice, 25 mice in each. The first group contained 10-week-old mice to serve as a control for normal response. The second group were old mice aged 22 months. Then we injected them with a foreign antigen to measure their immune response. The young control group produced almost 300 units of antibody against the antigen. By comparison the old mice only managed to produce 130 units of antibody.

This proved to us that a CoQ deficiency together with the

CHART B

Modification of Coenzyme Q Deficiency Index in Thymus and Body, Liver, Spleen, and Thymus Weight in Old Mice

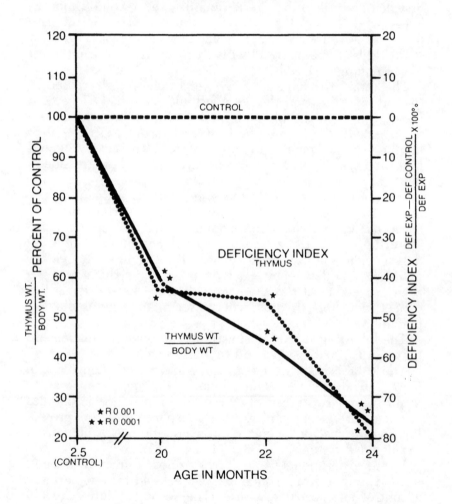

reduction in thymus weight results in a highly significant impairment of immune capability as evaluated in our experiments by measuring antibody levels. Could CoQ restore the depressed immune function in these old animals?

A third group of old mice (aged 22 months) were injected with a single injection of Coenzyme Q_{10} (as indicated on the following, Chart C). The old mice responded with a vigorous antibody production, almost reaching the high level of young mice. After CoQ treatment they were able to produce a highly significant 250 units of antibody. Remember, this was the result of a single administration of CoQ.

This dramatic improvement is illustrated on Chart C.

Additional Confirmation

In late 1985 a biochemical research team from the University of Michigan published a scientific paper that further reinforced the belief that CoQ plays a crucial role in aging. The researchers from the Laboratory of Chemical Biology, Department of Cellular and Molecular Biology, in Ann Arbor, studied the decline in CoQ levels during the life spans of male laboratory rats. And their findings were to isolate the heart, kidneys, and skeletal muscles as specifically showing significant reduction of CoQ during the aging process.

A report on the work stated, "The coenzyme Q (ubiquinone) concentrations of a number of tissues have been determined over the life span of the male laboratory rat. Coenzyme Q increased between 2 and 18 months and decreased significantly at 25 months in the heart and kidney, and the gastrocnemius, oblique and deep aspect (red) vastus lateralis muscles." It concluded that the cellular diminution of CoQ "may contribute to the loss of cellular function accompanying aging."

These findings once more help to confirm the importance of maintaining adequate levels of CoQ, and that these levels decline seriously with aging, thus threatening the entire bioenergetic capabilities at the cellular level, especially in major organs like the heart and kidneys.

The mechanism of aging is infinitely complicated, but new discoveries offer fascinating insights into some of the reasons at the most basic chemical levels.

CHART C

Increased Antibody Response (Hemolytic Units) after a Single
Administration of CoQ

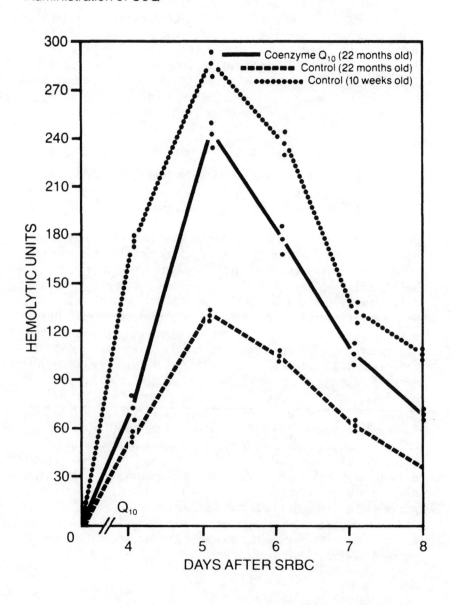

Free Radicals

Free radicals are very much the vogue in life-extension circles. As a term, it is bandied about loosely, mainly by practitioners in the nutrition and health fields, as the ultimate reason for all the ills of aging—consequently anything that counters free radicals has got to aid in the fight against aging. Yet few people actually know what free radicals are, and how they figure in the process of aging.

There is little doubt that free radicals may indeed contribute a crucial aspect to the dilemmas of advancing age. The National Institute on Aging (NIA) considers the role of free radicals in aging to be of such importance that the Institute states:

> Many of the conditions prevalent in later life—rheumatoid arthritis, cancer, and serious infections—are thought to occur because immunological responsiveness changes with old age. One age-related alteration in the immune system is the decrease in lymphocyte [white blood cells] response to antigens [foreign substances which may initiate disease]. A possible factor contributing to the decline in lymphocyte function is free radical damage. Free radicals are unstable chemical fragments that readily react with—and thus sometimes damage—other molecules. Some scientists contend that, although free radicals are normally cleared from the body without causing functional damage and some free radical reactions are beneficial, an age-related accumulation of such damage may ultimately interfere with the vital functioning of cell structures.

The NIA notes that its studies to determine whether the age-related decline in the immune system is partially the result of free radical damage to lymphocytes, are of paramount importance. And it adds, "It is possible that, in the future, antioxidants may be used to maintain immune function and thus reduce the degree of illness in the elderly."

The importance of CoQ in the free radical scenario figures in the fact that free radicals can be neutralized by antioxidants, and CoQ is a powerful antioxidant.

What Exactly Are Free Radicals?

Free radicals are renegade molecules circulating throughout the body. And it has been shown that they become more prolific as we age.

The free radical theory in aging is relatively new—only a couple of decades old. But it has helped increase our understanding of aging and may explain how some of our killer diseases get their start. Free radicals have been implicated in everything from heart disease, hardening of the arteries, arthritis, cancer, allergies, and even dandruff, as well as the aging process in general.

A free radical starts out life as a normal molecule. When atoms come together to create molecules they are bonded together by electron bridges, which attach them at two points. These electron bridges always occur in pairs, and this is the natural way that all molecules are formed in the body.

But sometimes the molecular bonds disintegrate and the two electron bridges that attached them are broken. Under normal circumstances this is no problem if they break off in equal pairs—but a free radical is created when a single electron bridge remains attached to one molecule, and its electron twin departs, attached to another molecule.

A unique situation of only one electron on each molecule has occurred. This makes them incompatible for further bonding with other "healthy" molecules that have two normal electrons. To make things even worse, the renegade molecules are highly active and unstable. They continue hunting for other molecules from which they can steal a second electron. Of course, when that happens their victim also becomes a free radical. Free radicals may propagate through hundreds of thousands of molecules before they bump into another free radical and neutralize each other. They don't have any particular goal, leading only a haphazard existence as destructive forces within the body's molecular chemistry.

The frightening prospect is that free radicals can continue creating other free radicals out of "healthy" molecules if they remain unchecked. Millions of otherwise normal molecules, serving vital functions in the body, can be totally disrupted by just a handful of free radicals.

This can have disastrous effects, for example when free radicals damage the DNA and RNA molecules in the cell nucleus—leading to mutant cells, which may result in cancerous cells. Another example might involve cells of the immune system that simply don't replicate themselves exactly as they should, leading to ineffective defenses.

Fortunately we have fail-safe mechanisms, natural checks and balances, to correct this unwanted phenomenon. Nature is able to scavenge free radicals by offering them more attractive but less important targets. Natural free radical scavengers have extra available electrons which they can sacrifice without damage. Many of these scavengers are closely related molecules that contain sulfur, selenium, and trace metals like copper, zinc, and manganese.

Free radical scavengers are known to include vitamin E, vitamin C, vitamin A, and beta-carotene (provitamin A), as well as coenzyme Q. Many of these scavengers may not always be present in optimal amounts in the body, due to malnutrition or aging for example. It is known that the availability of CoQ declines with age and that the formation of free radicals increases.

Antioxidants

Free radicals can be released as an unwanted by-product of a naturally occurring process in the body called lipid peroxidation, or, in simpler terms, fat oxidation resulting in fatty acids. This process is one of the most widely known and best understood and is known to accelerate aging. The free radicals are, in essence, unwanted and dangerous oxygen molecules or peroxides (molecules containing a harmful excess of oxygen).

CoQ has the ability to manipulate oxygen. It can add or take away oxygen from a given biochemical combination, moving oxygen in or out of the mitochondria. It can increase oxygen levels when necessary, and reduce them if they threaten to reach toxic levels.

Consequently, CoQ performs as an antioxidant by removing excess molecules of oxygen when they pose a danger. CoQ can therefore have the ability to neutralize the free radical oxygen renegades. Free radicals damage the protective membranes of cells and their inner mitochondria. Once inside, they can disrupt the delicate chemical balance within the inner sanctums of cells, damaging DNA and RNA in the cell's nucleus, which can in turn lead to incorrectly manufactured proteins.

Knowing that the immune system instantly recognizes anything foreign to the body—as would be the case of wrongly manufactured proteins—it swings into action to dispense with these "invaders." The proliferation of free radicals increases with age, and this can cause a tremendous drain on the immune system's natural resources. The immune system that was once perfectly capable of combatting illness, may now become so exhausted with this extra workload and the eventual cellular damage resulting from the free radicals, that it is unable to fight off diseases—the same disease states we associate with aging!

Another factor comes into play here. The exhausted immune system may also become totally confused and unable to distinguish between proteins that are native to the body and the proteins of genuine invaders, such as bacteria, viruses, and even cancer cells. The result is that the body's own defense system actually turns against itself. This is known as autoimmune disease—some forms of which are also very common in old age.

Now it becomes easier to visualize the crucial link between the immune system and aging. Clearly, without the protection of antioxidants, the runaway effect of free radicals could eventually take over the whole body—a domino effect resulting in an endless sequence of biochemical functions going wrong in a chain reaction that will eventually lead to death.

CoQ as a Potent Antioxidant

We already know that CoQ works at or on the mitochondria levels of the cell. It is most likely here that its important action as an antioxidant takes place. At the mitochondria level it can encounter a free radical and neutralize it before it has a chance to endanger any other vital biological processes by disrupting the delicate chemical balance.

CoQ researcher Dr. Lars Ernster of the Department of Biochemistry at the University of Stockholm, Sweden, makes an interesting observation. He points out, "It may be important to notice that many of the pathological conditions in which beneficial effects of ubiquinone have been described are among those where oxygen toxicity due to free radical formation has been implicated."

Dr. Ernster has listed clinically important situations in which oxygen radicals may play a significant role in tissue injury. They include:

• Chemotherapeutic agents: Adriamycin, streptozotocin, bleomycin
  • Myocardial infarction (heart attack—infarct size)
  • Cardiopulmonary bypass (heart bypass)

- Organ preservation and transplantation
- Stress ulcers
- Intestinal ischemia (lack of oxygen to gut tissues)
- Postshock hepatic (liver) failure
- Cerebral (brain) ischemia
- Limb ischemia
- Limb reimplantation
- Neutrophil phagocytosis (immune response)
- Arthritis
- Inflammatory bowel disease
- Connective tissue diseases (lupus)
- Immune deficiencies
- Aging
- Circulatory shock
- Peripheral edema (retention of fluids)

Dr. Ernster continues,

"It is striking to see that many of these disorders—adriamycin toxicity; ischemia/reperfusion syndromes including myocardial infarction, postshock hepatic failure and cerebral ischemia; inflammatory disorders, including connective tissue diseases and immune deficiencies; circulatory shock, aging—are among those in which therapeutic effects of ubiquinone administration have been reported.

"Ubiquinone may exert these effects by acting as an antioxidant, similar to vitamin E. In fact, there is evidence for a protective effect of ubiquinone against lipid peroxidation . . . which results in serious membrane damage and is also responsible for the deposition of granules found in aging cells ('age granules'). It is counteracted by antioxidants such as ubiquinone."

Dr. G. Lenaz and Dr. G. Parenti Castelli of the Botanical Institute and Institute of Biochemistry, in Bologna, Italy, report, "Evidence is accumulating that Q may act as an antioxidant. Studies in isolated mitochondria support the view that the reduced form of Q exhibits antioxidant effects, preventing the formation of lipid peroxides." The scientists added that new research strongly suggests that CoQ is a highly active neutralizer of free radicals.

In their very latest research, published in 1985, Lenaz and

Parenti Castelli further confirm their findings of CoQ's vital role in quenching dangerous free radicals. But they make the extremely significant point that while we may need CoQ for counteracting free radicals, it is also supremely vital for the regular bioenergetics of cellular energy, and as age and the proliferation of free radicals increase, our supplies of CoQ may be spread dangerously thin.

The calls on CoQ with the advancement of the aging process may indeed put the body in a situation of biological double jeopardy. Comments Dr. Lenaz, "It must be recalled that Q plays other roles in cells, besides its bioenergetic function; for example, it was shown to be a potent antioxidant agent. It can be speculated that an increased need, e.g. for antioxidant activity and scavenging of free radicals, could divert Q from its use in the respiratory chain and make its redox function insufficient." This observation further emphasizes the potential importance of taking supplemental daily oral dosages of CoQ as age advances.

Yet another important role of CoQ as an antioxidant has been reported to Dr. G. P. Littarru of the Institute of Biological Chemistry and Clinical Chemistry, in Rome, Italy, and it provides a significant clue as to what the reason may be for CoQ's action being so beneficial in protecting the heart during major surgery.

It is known that hypoxia, or lack of oxygen, can lead to tissue damage and death of tissue cells. It has also been known for some years that when tissue is abused or injured, oxidants, which are harmful to our cells, are produced at the site of injury. This action may indeed be part of our natural inbuilt defense to ward off infections at the injury because, although oxidants are harmful to our own cells, they are also highly toxic to invading organisms.

In major heart surgery (or in any other major organ surgery) it is inevitable that blood supply to the organ has to be terminated for periods of time, and the resulting hypoxia can cause tissue damage. It is known that CoQ somehow buffers against the effects of hypoxia during surgical procedures.

Dr. Littarru suggests that this often lifesaving benefit of CoQ is a direct result of CoQ's ability to quench the dangerous oxidants being produced by the injured tissues as a result of hypoxia, thus significantly reducing the overall chances of permanent injury and even tissue death.

Are We Meant to Live Longer?

The simple answer may be no. But don't lose heart. There's a growing body of research to suggest that the decline in antioxidants and the proliferation of destructive free radicals is nature's own pruning to ensure that we don't outlive our biological and reproductive usefulness.

Most evidence now indicates that humans have evolved the biological capacity to maintain optimum vigor and health to an age of about 30 to 40 years. After that there's a rapid decline in physiological and mental maximum performance and an increase in the onset of disease. Particularly evident is the onset of a broad spectrum of diseases such as cancer after the age of 30 or 40 years.

Dr. Richard G. Cutler of the Gerontology Research Center, National Institute on Aging at Baltimore City Hospital, offers very good reasoning for why this 30 to 40 year limit should be so. He explains that it is part of the evolutionary basis for humans—and the only reason we are living into our 60s and 70s today is because of increased medical and health knowledge. He points out, "For instance, the mean life span for human populations up to about 400–500 years ago was about 30–40 years. The recent increase in mean life span to the present level of about 70 years was largely the result of lowered environmental hazards, a decrease in infectious diseases and better nutrition." Dr. Cutler also makes a good fundamental point by looking at the animal kingdom and noting that "few animals living in their natural ecological niche" ever live to a chronological age where they begin to suffer seriously from the disabling effects of aging. In other words, in their natural habitat you never expect to see an aged or infirm animal.

What this suggests is that humans are indeed living on borrowed time once they pass 40, and that the free radicals may be serving a biological purpose on an evolutionary level, to literally put an end to human life and spare the uncomfortable ravages of aging.

This theory also promotes the survival of the fittest (the most basic concept of evolution) to propagate future generations—while the old and infirm are weeded out by death so as not to be able to reproduce again, possibly bearing weaker strains of the human species. This does make sense, and it fits in with all the classical descriptions from the theory of evolution. Free radicals may well be one of the biological safety valves that ensures that elderly members of the species are not able to reproduce inferior models.

But there is another important evolutionary point. Evolution is exactly what it says—an ever evolving and changing biology. Whether it happens naturally over millions of years, or it is artificially induced in just one century, it is still the true process of evolution.

If we discover the capability to extend life, and more importantly the quality of life, by "fooling" the natural processes of aging, we might just be short-circuiting a process that would eventually have occurred naturally, without our present interference, a few thousand years down the road from now. It might be considered foolish of us not to take advantage of the newly developing knowledge that has enabled us to recognize the processes of aging and develop new exciting tools to alter the biological clock.

By manipulating one of the most basic processes of aging—counteracting the bio-destructive effects of free radicals with antioxidants like CoQ—it may be possible to extend the quality of existence to catch up with the quantity of life extension that has already been created by medical advances over the past century or so.

CHAPTER 15

•

AIDS: A Rationale for CoQ Therapy

No single killing disease state has instilled more panic in recent history than acquired immunodeficiency syndrome (also known as acquired immune deficiency syndrome or AIDS). Only the influenza pandemic of 1918, which resulted in the deaths of 20 million people around the world, can over-shadow the present threat of AIDS for high mortality rates.

As many as 1.5 to 2 million Americans may already have been exposed to the AIDS virus, and up to 10 percent of them could ultimately come down with the deadly disease. At present it is known that 14,500 people in this country are caught in a life-and-death struggle with AIDS. Public health officials believe that of the people who have already been exposed to AIDS, some 75 percent may never experience any illness. But they may pass the virus to individuals who could eventually develop a full-blown AIDS state. And this is where a weak immune system could make a critical difference.

What is so frightening about AIDS is its potential to thrive unchecked, not only in one minority segment of the population, but to spread unhalted throughout society without a cure being found. The number of new cases of AIDS contin-ues to double about every 10 months. A vaccine to combat AIDS is not expected, even optimistically, much before 1990.

When it was first recognized in 1981, AIDS came as a surprise. Many disease specialists admit that society had de-luded itself into believing that diseases of epidemic propor-tions were a thing of past history. Bubonic plague, smallpox, and malaria had been controlled, and in most senses elimi-nated, by the astute work of biological detectives and newly developed vaccines, drugs, and antibiotics.

What caused the recognition of AIDS to pass from surprise to shock in the medical community was the realization that a new strain of virus had apparently come out of nowhere, or developed unnoticed, in not just a few isolated cases, but, as investigators were soon to learn, an entire subpopulation.

Origins

AIDS has surprising parallels with syphilis, another mainly sexually transmitted disease that was first brought to Europe by members of Columbus's crews who contracted it from Indians in the Americas.

Syphilis was a mysterious and devastating disease because it appeared unstoppable. It did, in fact, return in force back to its native land a century or so later. Syphilis has been controlled, but it still remains a disease of public health significance in the United States, accounting for 80,000 new cases each year, according to the National Institute of Allergy and Infectious Diseases.

It is believed that AIDS may have had its viral roots in Africa, where it might have been contained had it not been transferred somehow to the Americas where it has found a new breeding ground in a sexually liberal society. Its path might be said to have mirrored syphilis in reverse.

A fatal disease in Africa, known as "slim disease," has some striking similarities to AIDS. Only reported earlier this decade, slim disease shares many of the same symptoms as AIDS, but it is mainly characterized by extreme weight loss and it is transmitted predominantly among sexually promiscuous heterosexuals.

Medical scientists writing in the British journal *The Lancet* in 1985 reported that although slim disease resembles AIDS in so many ways, it appears to be a new entity—but the virus suspected of causing it may be a similar strain to that of AIDS.

Out of 71 patients recently diagnosed as suffering from slim disease, 63 showed evidence of infection with the AIDS virus. The puzzle here is why some patients show positive AIDS signs, and others do not.

Victims of slim disease are not likely to exhibit the swollen lymph glands and rare form of cancer called Kaposi sarcoma, both common features of AIDS. The first signs of slim disease are usually intermittent fevers and a general feeling of sickness, followed a month or so later by gradual, but unremitting, weight loss.

Researchers in the United States believe that slim disease may be yet another AIDS-related spin-off, or distant relative. AIDS-related complexes are known as ARC, a collection of conditions that are similar to the AIDS syndrome. Another disease similar to AIDS is called simian acquired immunodeficiency syndrome (SAIDS), which has only been found in monkeys.

What makes the discovery of these AIDS-like syndromes so intriguing is that the AIDS now recognized in our populations may not be as unique a virus as was originally believed.

Transmission

The AIDS virus is new in man. It is transmitted mainly in the semen, and mostly between homosexual men. It has been observed predominantly in homosexuals, Haitians, and by drug users who may share needles with victims who already carry the virus. Females can carry the disease, but the proportion of them that might pass it on through normal sexual relationships is believed to be minute compared to male homosexual activity. Another obvious problem is that AIDS can be transmitted by blood transfusion or by certain other blood products, such as plasma. A number of unfortunate transfusion-related AIDS cases have been recorded. Because the unborn children of AIDS infected mothers-to-be share the same blood system, a child can be born with AIDS.

Researchers discovered the AIDS virus in other body fluids, such as tears and saliva, and this gave rise to fears that it could be transmitted by simple forms of social contact. Studies now show that people who have had long-term and affectionate contact (including kissing) with AIDS victims may exhibit no signs of the virus having been transmitted to them.

There was also the discovery that people can carry AIDS antibodies without displaying any symptoms of the disease. It must be understood that the presence of AIDS antibodies does not show that a person presently has AIDS. What it does mean is that at some point in time he or she has been exposed to the AIDS virus, and the immune system has recognized the situation and through its natural defenses has produced antibodies against the AIDS invader. But it also suggests a likelihood that the person with AIDS antibodies may have a greater chance—than a person without the presence of AIDS antibodies—of developing the disease. The

AIDS virus may be somehow lying dormant within his or her body.

The symptoms of AIDS may include fever, night sweats, swollen glands in the neck, armpits, or groin (all glands of the immune system), unexplained weight loss, oral yeast infections, diarrhea, persistent coughs, fatigue, and loss of appetite.

Full-blown AIDS totally destroys the competence of the immune system, leaving a person particularly susceptible to pneumonia, Kaposi sarcoma, a rarer form of cancer of the blood vessel walls, and a myriad of other opportunist infections.

A Unique Virus

The AIDS virus is unlike any other previously encountered. AIDS belongs to a group called retroviruses. It has been named HTLV-III.

Regular viruses, like the ones that cause colds and flu, are made up of DNA (deoxyribonucleic acid), the genetic blueprints and building blocks found in all living things. Once a virus penetrates a cell it commandeers part of the cell's manufacturing machinery to make more clones of itself. Eventually the cell ruptures and these newly formed viruses swarm out to infect yet more healthy cells. As this process continues the immune system swings into full attack. With a cold, for example, this results in sniffles, fatigue, and symptoms like sinus and chest congestion, as antibodies and the other defense mechanisms are called into play to defeat the invading viruses.

A virus is only beaten when its chain of reproduction is halted, and this brings an end to the infection. But with the AIDS virus the immune scenario is different. Retroviruses like AIDS are far more dangerous. They are composed of RNA (ribonucleic acid), and the retrovirus utilizes the same cellular machinery to replicate copies of itself. Then it goes one stage further and incorporates this genetic knowledge into DNA's genetic structure to become part of the cell's permanent genetic code. The viral DNA sends out messages to make more retroviruses.

The cycle goes unbroken in retroviruses like AIDS. Thus it becomes a lifelong infection. The AIDS viruses make their homes in the T cells of the immune system, the very same frontline fighters intended to obliterate a viral adversary. As the virus takes over these key immune system cells, it effectively becomes a killer by suppressing the actions of the lymphocytes, leaving the body open to all kinds of opportunistic infections, including rare cancers not normally associated with a strong immune system.

Latest Anti-AIDS Drugs and CoQ

Developing drugs that will be effective against the virus associated with AIDS is an overwhelming challenge, but progress is already being made.

Many scientists believe it may be almost impossible to produce an agent capable of totally destroying the AIDS virus in the body, because of its unusual resilience. Drugs that might have the power to destroy the virus would also kill valuable T cells in detrimental quantities. A drug that could halt, or retard, the progress of the AIDS virus is most likely as close as science will get to eliminating it in the immediate future.

Early so called breakthroughs in AIDS research clearly illustrate the difficulty in finding an effective treatment. One example was the treatment developed by three doctors at the Laennec Hospital in Paris in late 1985. It involved the use of the well-known immunosuppressant cyclosporine, a drug that is used successfully to retard immune reaction and rejection in situations like organ transplantation. The researchers reported "spectacular" improvements in two AIDS patients, one of whom was considered close to death, who were treated with cyclosporine for 5 days. The researchers theorized that the cyclosporine treatment deactivated the immune system, and, strangely, in turn allowed the critical T cells to regenerate while the AIDS virus, presumably, was also being laid low.

Within a matter of days of the announcement of the "breakthrough," the French were reporting that not one, or two, but three AIDS victims undergoing treatment with cyclosporine had died. One 27-year-old male had been treated with cyclosporine for only 6 days before his death, and one of the victims had died after only 2 days on the drug, even before the breakthrough was called to the attention of the world.

But at the prestigious Weizmann Institute in Israel, researchers announced in 1985 yet another breakthrough, this time involving a hormone as a possible treatment for AIDS. Tests involving AIDS victims showed partial recovery of their immune systems, and at least one patient had been released from the hospital and described as in "remission." This was to be the first time claims were made that an AIDS victim's disease was even partially reversed.

The Israeli researchers reported that the hormone was a thymic humoral factor (THF) found in minute quantities in the human thymus gland. As stated in Chapter 3, the thymus, after puberty, disappears almost altogether, yet it is believed to play a key role in the cellular immunological response.

Thymus factors are a new development in medicine. Lost function of the thymus has been replaced by various factors isolated from healthy thymuses, or synthesized in the laboratory. Thus the ability exists to replace the lost function; a similar practice, for example, to giving insulin to the diabetic.

In our own research with animal models we discovered that levels of CoQ in the thymus, and the gland's size and weight, decline at exactly the same rate with age. But when supplemental CoQ was administered, increased immune response associated with the thymus was greatly restored, almost to the point of youthful immune response. If this avenue of approach, utilizing thymic factors, is proven to be of benefit in combatting AIDS, it strongly suggests a rationale for utilizing CoQ to boost thymus, and therefore immune, efficiency.

The National Institute of Allergy and Infectious Diseases, part of the National Institutes of Health, recently described four anti-AIDS agents presently in Phase I clinical trials. These are suramin, ribavirin, the French agent HPA-23, and azidothymidine. Of these, azidothymidine (previously known in research circles as Compound S), now called AZT, has shown to be the most promising. The beneficial action of AZT has surprising parallels with the already proven benefits of CoQ on the immune system, and especially the T cells.

CoQ has been shown to enhance phagocytosis (killer-scavenger cells) in the immune system, and to reverse cellular immunosuppression, probably by correcting a distorted ratio of T to B cells. Researchers from Burroughs Welcome Co, Duke University School of Medicine, The National Cancer Institute, and Memorial Sloan-Kettering Cancer Center attempted to elucidate the similar phagocytic mode of action of AZT against retroviruses, the same viral family to which HTLV-III belongs.

Studies showed that when AZT is added to a culture of T-helper lymphocytes infected with the AIDS virus, the killing effects of HTLV-III are blocked. It is the killing of T-helper lymphocytes that causes the characteristically reduced helper T cell to suppressor T cell ratio. This leaves the AIDS victim predisposed to life-threatening opportunistic infections such as pneumonia.

It has already been proved that CoQ displays a powerful action in animal model studies to boost the effect of lymphocytes and other cells of the immune system against deadly infectious agents. Although still speculation, the connection does seem obvious between the proven immune boosting benefits of CoQ and the type of immune boosting being sought in AIDS research and therapy.

The already displayed and scientifically recorded beneficial effects of CoQ on the animal and human immune system, and especially its probable role in promoting helper T cells, clearly show that the addition of CoQ, possibly as an adjunct to AIDS therapy, may yet add another powerful biomedical weapon to help fight this disease.

Latest major medical evaluations of the progress in AIDS research (taking place at The International Conference on AIDS, June, 1986, in Paris; and the 6th International Congress of Immunology, July, 1986, in Toronto, Canada) revealed a dim future for the development of effective AIDS therapy. An evaluation by the *American Medical News*, an organ of the American Medical Association covering these two important meetings, agreed that the future for a breakthrough in AIDS therapy was extremely pessimistic.

A surprise presentation by a Soviet scientist at the Paris meeting acknowledged the existence of AIDS cases over a long period of time in the USSR—further reinforcing the view that the problem of AIDS is a worldwide epidemic not just confined to "the decadent capitalistic society."

Note: A subcommittee empowered by the International Committee on Taxonomy of Viruses proposed, in a letter to *Science* (published in the issue of May 9, 1986), that the AIDS causing viruses be officially designated as the human immunodeficiency viruses, to be known in abbreviated form as HIV.

CHAPTER 16

•

CoQ: The Future

As an increasing number of CoQ's exciting benefits are continually being discovered and verified, it could be expected that Coenzyme Q_{10} might one day become as regularly used as aspirin and vitamin C.

In Japan new CoQ drugs are constantly being developed. One of the very latest CoQ drugs to be introduced to the Japanese market is an antiulcer compound that utilizes an early discovery made by ubiquinone researchers; CoQ's ability to protect gastric tissues.

Some of the impressive new CoQ research being pursued not only includes CoQ and the immune system—with diseases like diabetes, muscular dystrophy, multiple sclerosis, and lupus erythematosus—it also involves CoQ's beneficial role involving allergies, asthma and respiratory disease states, and the brain with the potential benefits of treating anomalies of mental function, like schizophrenia, and even Alzheimer's disease.

AIDS is a primary target for CoQ research. CoQ's immense beneficial potential involving the immune system cannot be ignored. Another aspect also being investigated by Japanese scientists is the administration of CoQ by targeting it to specific organs and systems in the body. Yet another area of research is the possibility of developing a simple blood test that would measure levels of CoQ in the entire body.

Much of the future studies involving CoQ will depend on the actions of the FDA. If it is classified as a prescription drug, as it is already in Japan, this will give added impetus to the Western pharmaceutical companies to produce their own versions of CoQ, and give a boost to its present availability.

Here is a look at some of the new horizons involving CoQ.

A CoQ Test

The health implications from one individual blood sampling of CoQ are very exciting. Accurate measurements of blood levels of CoQ are already available to ubiquinone researchers. The process is presently time-consuming and costly as only a few laboratories are equipped to perform this function. But as the demand for CoQ testing grows, this situation will change rapidly. It can be expected that a simple test initiated in the physician's office will be all that is necessary for determination of CoQ levels in the near future.

A small blood sample drawn by the physician, or even a small tissue sample, would then be sent away to be processed by a biochemical laboratory specialized in CoQ analysis. The report the physician receives back will enable him to determine not only overall health (how well a variety of organs are performing, such as the heart, liver, immune system), but also to pinpoint potential trouble.

Among the areas he will be able to observe are

- Overall CoQ level.
- General health.
- A deficiency of CoQ.

By combining the initial analysis with more specific tests he will be able to determine

- How well the heart and other organs are performing.
- How well the immune system is functioning.
- Whether the effects of any existing medications may benefit from the addition of CoQ as an adjunct therapy.
- Whether CoQ may aid in reducing potential toxic side effects of existing, or proposed, medications.
- If CoQ may be justified for controlling existing conditions, like hypertension.
- Whether further investigation is needed into specific areas of health.

He might also be able to predict

- The onset of disease states, especially heart disease and cancer, that can be reflected in CoQ deficiency levels.
- The potential for immune system deficiencies and related problems.
- Whether CoQ taken prophylactically could avert impending ill health or disease states.

It soon becomes clear, when taking all these possibilities into consideration, that a simple test to determine overall levels of CoQ could one day be one of the most valuable tools available to the family physician as a diagnostic overview.

Of course in medicine no single test is accepted as one hundred percent accurate, and it would be important for a physician to make a judgment in conjunction with the results of other diagnostic tests appropriate to any condition indicated by a CoQ deficiency. If it were suspected that a deficiency of CoQ may be contributing to increased incidences of infections, in an aging patient for example, further evaluations of immune system parameters, including immunoglobulin levels, T cell functions, and others, would then be appropriate to confirm a diagnosis.

Targeting CoQ

Magic bullets, drugs that can be shot to very specific targets in the human body, have always been the dream of drug developers.

There are a number of ways to target a drug, but one is to rely on the different rates of uptake between tissues in the human body and the affinity they have for different substances. For example, if you know the heart has an affinity for Compound X, while other organs don't, then Compound X might very well make a useful transport system to deliver a drug to the heart, and the heart only.

In very simple terms, you could encapsulate a heart drug in Compound X and enter it into the body. Knowing that Compound X will only be absorbed by the heart muscle, the drug can be delivered precisely. Once the outer coating of Compound X is broken down in the heart, the drug contained inside is released: simple, and very effective.

The possibility of targeting CoQ is now being studied by pharmaceutical companies in Japan. This system has some distinct advantages. Consider the problem of introducing 100 mg of CoQ orally for a known heart deficiency. How much of that CoQ is actually going to get into the heart? The answer is, unfortunately, only a small percentage. Other organs have a high affinity for CoQ, particularly the liver. If a way could be found to bind CoQ to another substance, which only the heart would absorb, it can be targeted direct with the assurance that the major part of the nutrient was going where it was needed.

Researchers have reported on the success of utilizing liposomes as carriers for the delivery of therapeutic and diagnostic agents to specific targets within the body. Liposomes, coated with a natural substance called amylopectin, were found to be readily taken up into the lung. Liposomes combined with sulfatide have been targeted directly to the brain. Now Japanese scientists are working on targeting CoQ to the heart.

These projects are so new that all that has been revealed at this time is that researchers are having success targeting to the heart by combining CoQ with a soy-lecithin microemulsion. Coenzyme Q as a magic bullet may be just around the corner.

Muscular Dystrophy

Muscular dystrophy is a group of inherited diseases characterized by progressive weakness and the degeneration of muscle fibers, without evidence of neural involvement. It has not been a strong focus of CoQ research, but Dr. Karl Folkers has studied a number of muscular dystrophy sufferers and reports some optimistic results.

The results of CoQ therapy for muscular dystrophy are somewhat confusing: Dr. Mineharu Sugimoto, of Kumamoto University Medical School, in Japan, studied over 50 patients with various forms of neuromuscular diseases, especially dystrophy, and he could find no significant beneficial effects among those patients treated with CoQ. But he admitted that unlike the reported successes by Dr. Folkers and others, he had used much smaller doses of CoQ, only 45 mg a day compared to 250 mg to 1 gm a day by Folkers and others.

"Folkers used larger doses. Accordingly our dosage of administration appears to be low in comparison to others. In this connection, Folkers proposed that dystrophy represents a CoQ_{10} dependency state which should require much larger amounts of CoQ_{10}," says Dr. Sugimoto.

Dr. Folkers also advocated catching the disease state early for CoQ treatment. By comparison, the Japanese studies involved intermediate and late stage patients, and the difference between the success noted by Folkers and the lack of success reported by Japanese researchers may hinge on this fact.

Individual case histories, presented by Dr. Folkers and coresearcher Dr. James Couch, do show promise. Dr. Folkers tells the following interesting story about one of his first involvements with CoQ and muscular dystrophy.

> Over six years ago, an adult with late onset form of muscle disease contacted me to volunteer to join our research program as a patient, because he had been advised by his neurologist that he should mentally prepare himself for a wheelchair within two years. Eight months or so after this medical prediction, which devastated the morale of this lawyer, he was placed on CoQ_{10}. I have long turned to Dr. Couch for medical advice, and when he reviewed this case, he remarked that if this patient could be kept out of a wheelchair for five years, we might well take a greater interest in CoQ_{10} and muscular dystrophy. This patient has now been on CoQ_{10} for only a few days less than 6 years—not just 5 years. He not only is not in a wheelchair, but he swims, bowls, and plays golf frequently each week and conducts a vigorous business life in his legal profession.

It is agreed among CoQ researchers that the nutrient does show distinct promise for victims of muscular dystrophy. Large scale trials are now being suggested.

Multiple Sclerosis

Multiple sclerosis is a slowly progressing disease characterized by a degeneration in the brain and the spinal cord and resulting in multiple varied neurological symptoms, usually with remissions and exacerbations.

Some 250,000 Americans are afflicted by the disease of multiple sclerosis. In some, it produces only mild movement disorders, but in others it causes paralysis, loss of speech, and damage to vision and mental functions, depending on which brain and nerve cells it destroys.

Researchers recently discovered a new virus in blood and brain fluids from multiple sclerosis patients in Sweden and Key West, Florida. It is now believed that this virus might be one cause of the unexplained disease. The virus has not yet been identified, but it is similar to HTLV-I, a virus that causes an unusual form of human leukemia.

Genetic material from the new virus has been identified in T cells of the immune system by researchers at the Wistar

Institute, in Philadelphia, the National Cancer Institute, and the University of Miami, who made the discovery that was reported in the British scientific journal, *Nature*.

What makes this finding so intriguing when considering CoQ is that it suggests that a potential cure for multiple sclerosis may be found to involve the immune system. Knowing of CoQ's ability to boost the immunocompetence, and especially the activity of phagocytes and other cells of the immune system, it may be prudent to investigate the beneficial potential of CoQ therapy for multiple sclerosis sufferers.

An interesting point to note is that the HTLV-I virus is believed by some researchers to be in the same family of viruses as the AIDS virus, which has been named HTLV-III.

Alzheimer's Disease, Schizophrenia, and Lupus

Alzheimer's is the disease of aging that we associate with increasing loss of memory and mental function. New research indicates that what was always referred to as senility—a not unexpected process of aging—may not be a result of longevity, but a distinct disease process in itself.

Schizophrenia is a psychotic disorder associated with behavioral and intellectual disturbances. Lupus is a complicated disease of unknown cause which can result in serious, often fatal, multiple afflictions of the joints, skin, kidney, heart, lungs, and brain.

What links these three disease states is a growing body of research that indicates they may result from a malfunction of the immune system. Viral infection is also suspected, and if this is proven to be so, the capabilities of a disordered immune system working at less than optimal efficiency could play a crucial role in how these diseases progress.

It is from this viewpoint that an approach to controlling any progression in Alzheimer's, schizophrenia, and lupus would be through restoring optimal immunocompetence to its fullest potential. It is already known that a serious deficiency of CoQ will result in a disordered immune system. In the case of these three particular disease states, a deficiency state could be the difference between why some people succumb to Alzheimer's, schizophrenia, or lupus, and others with no immune deficiencies don't.

In our own latest research among victims of lupus, the path we are following involves reviewing the malfunction of the immune system and the possible utilization of CoQ as a corrective therapy. It is too early yet to expect any practical results, but the hope is that CoQ will once more prove its immense value in the amelioration of yet more disease states.

Gastric Ulcers

An exciting new drug for sufferers of gastric and duodenal ulcers, or for that matter anybody who may be a high risk candidate for ulcers, is the latest CoQ preparation marketed by the Eisai Company of Japan.

The drug is called Teprenone (chemical name, geranyl-geranylacetone—or GGA) and is being sold under the trade name Selbex. It was first introduced to the pharmaceutical market in Japan in late 1984 as an antiulcer agent whose synthesis was inspired by the gastric protecting properties of CoQ. Early research involving CoQ reported that the nutrient appeared to demonstrate a protective action on the lining of the stomach and duodenum.

Contrary to popular myth, ulcers are not gastric eruptions, swellings, bumps or boils, but open sores, pits in the organ lining where the gastric juices have eaten through the membrane that normally protects the organ wall.

There can be many causes of gastric and duodenal ulcers, but bad eating habits combined with stress, which may produce an oversecretion of gastric acid, are usually the primary causes. Once the wound has been created, the healing process is extremely slow because the ulcer can be continually inflamed by the constant pumping of gastric juices into the digestive organs. This also creates the possibility of the ulcer growing as the gastric acid literally eats away at the exposed tissues of the organ wall.

Traditionally, solutions and tablets with high alkalinity (chalky compounds) are taken to neutralize the acidity of the digestive juices, thus providing a more helpful environment for the sore to heal. More modern therapy involves medicines that reduce gastric acid secretion.

During the first observations of CoQ's protective action, it was not fully understood how the nutrient was benefiting ulcer sufferers, although remarkable improvements were being observed. It is now believed that CoQ's action may be two-fold—working to improve the actual bioenergetics of the healing process, and promoting the enhancement of gastric mucosal glycoprotein (the secretion which normally lines and protects the organ walls from the gastric juices). If it was not for this protective process, the stomach and duodenum would quite literally be eaten alive by their own gastric acid in the same way that the acid breaks down meats and other food products.

Scientists at Eisai's laboratories in Gifu, Japan, examined the chemical structure of CoQ and, through painstaking elimination, narrowed down the curative benefits associated with ulcers to a portion of CoQ's polyprenyl side chain. They were then able to "snip" out this section of the molecule, study it, and synthesize it independently. The result: geranylgeranylacetone, or GGA, which forms the active basis of the new drug Selbex.

Experiments utilizing rats by Eisai researchers showed that GGA was indeed the potent section of the CoQ chain which best inhibited ulcers. They also discovered that GGA not only speeded up the healing process of induced ulcers in rats, but pretreatment with GGA before the induction of ulcers greatly inhibited their production.

In a 1981 paper, Dr. Manabu Murakami reported, "These results may suggest a high possibility that GGA is useful for clinical treatment of peptic ulcers, probably through a mechanism of increasing the defence force of the gastric mucosa."

Follow-up studies and clinical tests confirmed these early findings and Eisai was licensed to produce the CoQ "spin-off" as an antiulcer drug.

Allergy and Asthma

A fruitful area of research being pursued by CoQ investigators is the nutrient's ability to counter histamine and other mediator production, and this may prove to be of invaluable interest to allergy and asthma sufferers.

Allergy is an altered reaction, known as hypersensitivity, to a specific exogenous (outside-the-body) substance which causes no reaction in the nonsensitive individual. From the immunology point of view, allergy is an antibody-antigen reaction. The antigens, called allergens, may be molecules of protein, carbohydrate, lipid, or portions of those molecules. Known allergens are pollens, dust, moulds, poison ivy, bee stings, vaccines, serums, drugs, and a variety of other substances.

Of specific interest is allergic reactions to foods, common ones being eggs, milk, shrimp, grains, and even chocolate.

The clinical manifestations result from local or systemic (throughout the body) release of various highly active chemicals called mediators from tissue cells. These mediators are histamine, serotonin, prostaglandins, leukotriens, and others. Usually affected organs are the gastrointestinal tract, skin, and respiratory systems.

There are four types of allergic diseases:

1. *Anaphylaxis* is a pathological response induced by previous sensitization to a substance. In this group are allergies to some drugs and biological preparations (serums and vaccines).

2. *Atopy* is dependent upon an inherited constitutional capability. This group includes hay fever, rhinitis, asthma, skin eruptions in infants and adults, and some forms of drug sensitivity.

3. *Contact dermatitis* is a hypersensitivity to substances coming into contact with the skin.

4. *Serum sickness* is a hypersensitivity to injections of serum.

At the University of Tokyo, scientists have discovered that the introduction of CoQ can markedly decrease histamine release from lung tissue. Research reported in 1985 has shown that the activity which results in anaphylaxis is almost entirely triggered by leukotriens (also known as LTs) being released from the bronchial tissues.

The University of Tokyo researchers discovered LTs in the peripheral blood of patients undergoing attacks of bronchial asthma, and even found the substances in the lung fluids of patients with chronic bronchitis. In animal models they found that LTs induced potent contractile (coughing) responses in samples of tissue from the lungs of guinea pigs.

Previous research had reported that certain quinone derivatives with modified polyprenyl side chains had shown promise in inhibiting histamine, and LT, release. Consequently, the researchers decided to find out if CoQ might offer benefits. Using guinea pig lung tissue as a model they discovered that if the tissue was treated with CoQ before being exposed to the antigen, the levels of resulting LT production from the tissue could be greatly reduced.

The significance of this finding is extremely exciting. Immediate administration of CoQ might prove to be an ideal remedy for aborting asthmatic or allergic attacks, and even more important, long-term use of CoQ prophylactically may prevent attacks.

The report from the Tokyo researchers concluded, "Our results suggest that Coenzyme Q_{10} or its derivatives might become effective drugs against various kinds of obstructive lung diseases including bronchial asthma and anaphylactic shock."

In this book it is hoped that the reader may have marveled at the range of CoQ's beneficial potential, from its actions in bolstering the immune system to reversals in the most serious stages of terminal heart disease. The authors feel it is a fitting tribute to CoQ to have finished this last chapter with research displaying new hope of a natural remedy for alleviating the miserable histamine-produced symptoms in allergies and asthma, and possibly of man's most often suffered malady—the common cold.

And we make no apologies for closing with a repeat; a quote which appeared in the Introduction.

New and revolutionary treatments of disease, particularly where there has been no treatment of intrinsic biochemical significance, have generally been believable to a few persons and unbelievable and even ridiculous to others before proof of efficacy. I once heard the story of how incredible the first sulfur drug was to the treatment of infection. To treat pneumonia with a chemical was not considered sane. I witnessed the birth of cortisone to treat disease in a medical environment that was substantially unbelieving. Chemists, in conflict with influential medical opinion, solved the advent of vitamin B_{12}. Revolutionary therapy has always been so and perhaps always shall be, for such is the nature of true discovery. It appears that the bioenergetics of CoQ_{10} is remarkable and its potential in medicine is no exception to the history of controversial advances in medicine.

—Karl Folkers, Ph.D., 1981.

References

Aomine, Masahiro and Arita, Makoto. Isotachophoretic Evidence for Energy-Preservating Effect of Coenzyme Q_{10} on Isolated Guinea-Pig Cardiac Muscle. *General Pharmacology,* Vol. 15, No. 2, pp. 145–148, 1984.

————. Pretreatment with Coenzyme Q_{10} Protects Guinea Pig Ventricular Muscle from Hypoxia-Induced Deterioration of Action Potentials and Contraction. *General Pharmacology,* Vol. 16, No. 2, pp. 91–96, 1985.

Aubel-Sadron, Genevieve, and Londos-Galiardi, Danielle. Daunorubicin and Doxorubicin, Anthracycline Antibiotics, A Physicochemical and Biological Review. *Biochimie* 66 pp. 333–352, 1984.

Awata, Nobuhisa; Ishiyama, Taro; Harada, Hisato; et al. The Effects of Coenzyme Q_{10} on Ischemic Heart Disease Evaluated by Dynamic Exercise Test. *Biomedical and Clinical Aspects of Coenzyme Q,* Vol. 2. Elsevier/North-Holland Biomedical Press, 1980.

Azuma, I.; Sugimura, K.; Yamamura, M.; et al. The Effect of Ubiquinone-7 and Its Metabolites on the Immune Response. *International Journal for Vitamin and Nutrition Research* 48, No. 3, pp. 255–261, 1978.

Azuma, J.; Harada, H.; Sawamura, A.; et al. Beneficial Effect of Coenzyme Q on Myocardial Slow Action Potentials in Hearts Subjected to Decreased Perfusion Pressure-Hypoxia-Substrate-Free Perfusion. *Basic Research in Cardiology* 80, pp. 147– 155, 1985.

Baker, Lee E. "Gold Standards" and Impedance Cardiography. *Biomedical and Clinical Aspects of Coenzyme Q,* Vol. 4, Elsevier Science Publishers B.V., 1984.

Beyer, Robert E.; Burnett, Bonnie-Ann; Cartwright, Kenneth J., et al. Tissue Coenzyme Q (Ubiquinone) and Protein Concentrations over the Life Span of the Laboratory Rat. *Mechanisms of Ageing and Development* 32, pp. 267–281, Elsevier Scientific Publishers Ireland Ltd., 1985.

Bliznakov. Control and Reversal of the Immunological Senescence. United States Patent #4,156,718, May 29, 1979.

———— and Casey, A.; and Premuzic, E. *Coenzymes Q: Stimulants of the Phagocytic Activity in Rats and Immune Response in Mice.* Experientia, Vol. 26, pp. 953–954, 1970.

————, Emile G. Suppression of Immunological Responsiveness in Aged Mice and Its Relationship with Coenzyme Q Deficiency. *Macrophages and Lymphocytes*, Part A., pp. 361–369, 1980.

————. Coenzyme Q in Experimental Infections and Neoplasia. *Biomedical and Clinical Aspects of Coenzyme Q*, pp. 73–83, Elsevier/North-Holland Biomedical Press, 1977.

————. Coenzyme Q, the Immune System and Aging. *Biomedical and Clinical Aspects of Coenzyme Q*, Vol. 3, pp. 311–323, Elsevier/North-Holland Biomedical Press, 1981.

————. Serotonin and Its Precursors as Modulators of the Immunological Responsiveness in Mice. *Journal Of Medicine*, Vol. 11, Nos. 2 & 3, pp. 81–105, 1980.

————. Restoration of Impaired Immune Functions in Aged Mice by Coenzyme Q. Proceedings of the 4th International Congress of Immunology, Paris, France, July 21–26, 1980.

————. Immunological Senescence in Mice and Its Reversal by Coenzyme Q_{10}. *Mechanisms of Ageing and Development* 7, pp. 189–197, Elsevier Sequoia S.A., Lusanne, 1978.

————. Coenzyme Q Deficiency in Aged Mice. *Journal Of Medicine*, Vol. 9, No. 4, pp. 337–346, 1978.

————. *Effect of Stimulation of the Host Defense System by Coenzyme Q_{10} in Debenzpyrene-Induced Tumors and Infection with Friend Leukemia Virus in Mice*. Proc. Nat. Acad. Sci. USA, Vol. 70, pp. 390–394, 1973.

Block, Lutz H.; Georgopoulos, Apostolos; Mayer, Peter; and Drews, Jurgen. Nonspecific Resistance to Bacterial Infections: Enhancement by Ubiquinone-8. *Journal of Experimental Medicine*, Vol. 148, pp. 1228–1240, November 1978.

Bougnoux, Philippe; Bonvini, Ezio; Stevenson, Henry C.; et al. Identification of Ubiquinone-50 as the Major Mathylated Nonpola Lipid in Human Monocytes. *The Journal of Biological Chemistry*, Vol. 258, No. 7, April 10, pp. 4339–4344, 1983.

Bradley, Bender S. B Lymphocyte Function in Aging. *Review of Biological Research in Aging*, Vol. 2, pp. 143–154, 1985.

Cahn, Jean, and Borzeix, Marie-Gilberte. The Effect of Ubiquinone 50 Over the Sub-Acute Phase of an Experimental Stroke in the Rat. *Biomedical and Clinical Aspects of Coenzyme Q*, Vol. 4, pp. 209–217, Elsevier Science Publishers B.V., 1984.

Cahn, Jean; Boreix, Marie-Gilberte; Angignard, Jean; et al. Possible Use of Coenzyme Q_{10} in Acute Cerebral Disease. *Biomedical and Clinical Aspects of Coenzyme Q*, Vol. 3, pp. 385–395, Elsevier/North-Holland Biomedical Press, 1981.

Casu, A.; Cottalasso, D.; Pronzato, U.M.; et al. Rapid Modification of Ubiquinone Behaviour in Rat Liver Golgi Apparatus Subfractions after Acute Ethanol Intoxication. *IRCS Medical Science* 12, pp. 382–383, 1984.

Casu, A.; Cottalasso, D.; Pronzato, M.A.; et al. Phospholipids, Vitamin A and Ubiquinone of the Golgi Apparatus Subfractions from Rat

Liver after Acute Ethanol Intoxication. *Experimental Pathology* 25, pp. 251–255, 1984.

Chernukhina, L.O.; Donchenko, G.V.; Zolotashko, O.M.; and Teplytska, L. Yu. Content of Ubiquinone and Ubichromenol in Rat Liver at Different Supply of Organism with Vitamin E. The A.V. Palladin Institute of Biochemistry, Academy of Sciences, Ukranian SSR, Kiev, February 2, 1976.

Chiba, Michio. A Protective Action of Coenzyme Q_{10} on Chlorpromazine-Induced Cell Damage in the Cultured Rat Myocardial Cells. *Japanese Heart Journal*, Vol. 25, No. 1, pp. 127–137, January 1984.

Choe, Jae Y.; Combs, Alan B.; and Folkers, Karl. Prevention by Coenzyme Q_{10} of the Electrocardiographic Changes Induced by Adriamycin in Rats. *Research Communications in Chemical Pathology and Pharmacology*, Vol. 23, No. 1, January 1979.

Combs, Alan B.; Faria, Duyen Troung; Leslie, Steven W.; and Bonner, Hugh W. Effect of Coenzyme Q_{10} on Adriamycin Induced Changes in Myocardial Calcium. *Biomedical and Clinical Aspects of Coenzyme Q*, Vol. 3, pp. 137–143, Elsevier/North-Holland Biomedical Press, 1981.

Combs, Alan B.; Choe, Jae Y.; Truong, Duyen H.; and Folkers, Karl. Reduction by Coenzyme Q_{10} of the Acute Toxicity of Adriamycin in Mice. *Research Communications in Chemical Pathology and Pharmacology*, Vol. 18, No. 3, November 1977.

Cortes, Engracio O.; Guota, Mohinder; Chou, Chia; et al. Adriamycin Cardiotoxicity: Early Detection by Systolic Time Interval and Possible Prevention by Coenzyme Q_{10}. *Cancer Treatment Reports*, Vol. 62, No. 6, pp. 887–891, June 1978.

Cutler, Richard G. Antioxidants and Longevity. Free Radicals in Molecular Biology, *Aging and Disease*. Raven Press, New York, 1984.

Donchenkc, H.V.; Dyadychiv, A.M.; and Vovnyanko, E.K. Change in the Content of Ubiquinone in Rat Tissues with a Higher Concentration of Vitamins A and E in an Organism. Institute of Biochemistry, Academy of Sciences, Ukranian SSR, Kiev, April 1972.

Drews, J. Immunostimulation: Clinical and Experimental Perspectives. Klin Wochenschr 62, pp. 254–264, 1984.

Drzewoski, Josef; Baker, Lee; Richardson, Philip; et al. Apparent Effectiveness of Coenzyme Q_{10} to Increase Cardiac Function. *Biomedical and Clinical Aspects of Coenzyme Q*, Vol. 3, pp. 223–227, Elsevier/North-Holland Biomedical Press, 1981.

Eisai Co, Ltd., Tokyo, Japan. Drug Information: Nuequinon Capsules. November 1981.

Ernster, Lars. Ubiquinone: Redox Coenzyme, Hydrogen Carrier, Antioxidant. *Biomedical and Clinical Aspects of Coenzyme Q*, Vol. 4, pp. 3–13, Elsevier Science Publishers B.V., 1984.

Ernster, Lars, and Nelson, Dean B. Functions of Coenzyme Q. *Biomedical and Clinical Aspects of Coenzyme Q*, Vol. 3, pp. 159–167, Elsevier/North-Holland Biomedical Press, 1981.

Ernster, Lars, and Schatz, Gottfried. Mitochondria: A Historical Review. *The Journal of Cell Biology*, Vol. 91, No. 3, Pt. 2, pp. 227–255, December 1981.

Eskew, Mary Lou; Scholz, R.W.; Reddy, C.C.; et al. Effects of Vitamin E and Selenium Deficiencies on Rat Immune Function. *Immunology* 54, pp. 173–180, 1985.

Fabris, N., and Mocchegiani. Endocrine Control of Thymic Serum Factor Production in Young-Adult and Old Mice. *Cellular Immunobiology* 91, pp. 325–335, 1985.

Fahy, Gregory M. Life Extension Benefits of Coenzyme Q_{10}. *Antiaging News*, Vol. 3, No. 7, pp. 74–78, July 1983.

Folkers, Karl. Chairman's Opening Remarks. *Biomedical and Clinical Aspects of Coenzyme Q*, Vol. 4, pp. xiii, Elsevier Science Publishers B.V., 1984.

Folkers, Karl. Chairman's Closing Remarks. *Biomedical and Clinical Aspects of Coenzyme Q*, Vol. 4, pp. 429–430, Elsevier Science Publishers B.V., 1984.

Folkers, Karl; Baker, Lee; Richardson, Philip C.; et al. New Progress on the Biomedical and Clinical Research on Coenzyme Q. *Biomedical and Clinical Aspects of Coenzyme Q*, Vol. 3, pp. 399–412, Elsevier/ North-Holland Biomedical Press, 1981.

Folkers, Karl; Baker, Lee; Richardson, Philip C.; et al. On the Biomedical and Clinical Research on Coenzyme Q. *Biomedical and Clinical Aspects of Coenzyme Q*, Vol. 3, pp. 399–412, Elsevier/North-Holland Biomedical Press, 1981.

Folkers, K.; Littarru, G.P.; Nakamura, R.; and Scholler, J. Survey and New Clinical Studies on Coenzyme Q in Human Muscular Dystrophy. *International Journal of Vitamin and Nutritional Research* 42, pp. 140–163, 1972.

Folkers, Karl; Sartori, Michele; Baker, Lee; and Richardson, Philip C. Observations of Significant Reductions of Arrhythmias in Treatment with Coenzyme Q_{10} of Patients Having Cardiovascular Disease. *IRCS Medical Science* 10, pp. 348–349, 1982.

Folkers, Karl; Shizukuishi, Satoshi; Takemura, Kinzo; et al. Increase in Levels of IgG in Serum of Patients Treated with Coenzyme Q_{10}. *Research Communications in Chemical Pathology and Pharmacology*, Vol. 38, No. 2, November 1982.

Folkers, Karl; Vadhanavikit, Surasi; and Mortensen, Svend A. Biochemical Rationale and Myocardial Tissue Data on the Effective Therapy of Cardiomyopathy with Coenzyme Q_{10}. *Proc. Natl. Acad. Sci.* Vol. 62, pp. 901–904, February 1985.

Folkers K., and Wolaniuk, A. Research on Coenzyme Q_{10} in Clinical Medicine and in Immunomodulation. *Drugs under Experimental and Clinical Research*, Vol. 11, No. 8, pp. 539–546, 1985.

Folkers K., and Wolaniuk, A. Progress in Biomedical and Clinical Research on Coenzyme Q_{10}. *Drugs Experimental Clinical Research* X(7), pp. 513–517, 1984.

Folkers, Karl; Wolaniuk, Anna; Vadhanavikit, Surasi; et al. Biomedical and Clinical Research on Coenzyme Q_{10} with Emphasis on Cardiac Patients. *Biomedical and Clinical Aspects of Coenzyme Q*, Vol. 4, pp. 375–389, Elsevier Science Publishers B.V., 1984.

Furuta, Tatsuji; Kodama, Itsuo; Kondo, Noriaki; et al. A Protective Affect of Coenzyme Q_{10} on Isolated Rabbit Ventricular Muscle under Hypoxic Condition. *Journal of Cardiovascular Pharmacology* 4, pp. 1062–1067, 1982.

Graziano, Frank M., and Bell, Carolyn L. The Normal Immune Response and What Can Go Wrong. *Symposium on Clinical Immunology I*. Medical Clinics of North American, Vol. 69, No. 3, pp. 439–452, May 1985.

Hamada, Mareomi; Kazatani, Yukio; Ochi, Takaaki; et al. Correlation between Serum CoQ_{10} Level and Myocardial Contractility in Hypertensive Patients. *Biomedical and Clinical Aspects of Coenzyme Q*, Vol. 4, pp. 263–270, Elsevier Science Publishers B.V., 1984.

Heinzerling, Rollin H.; Tengerdy, Robert P.; Wick, Linda L.; and Lueker, David C. Vitamin E Protects Mice against Diplococcus Pneumoniae Type I Infection. *Infection and Immunity*, pp. 1292–1295, December 1974.

Hiasa, Yoshikazu; Ishida, Takatoshi; Maeda, Toshihiro; et al. Effects of Coenzyme Q_{10} on Exercise Tolerance in Patients with Stable Angina Pectoris. *Biomedical and Clinical Aspects of Coenzyme Q*, Vol. 4, pp. 291–300, Elsevier Science Publishers B.V., 1984.

Honjo, K.; Tsukamoto, Y.; Nakamura, R.; et al. Effect of Coenzyme Q_7 on Citric Acid Metabolism in Scurvy. *Archives of Oral Biology*, Vol. 11, pp. 543–546, Pergamon Press Ltd., 1966.

Igarashi, Toshiji; Nakajima, Yoshikage; Tanaka, Mamoru; and Ohtake, Shinzaburo. Effect of Coenzyme Q_{10} on Experimental Hypertension in Rats and Dogs. *The Journal of Pharmacology and Experimental Therapeutics*, Vol. 189, No. 1, pp. 149–156, 1974.

Imai, Shoichi; Tamatsu, Hirokuni; Ushijima, Toyohiko; et al. Effects of CoQ_{10} on Myocardial Energy Metabolism in Ischemia. *Biomedical and Clinical Aspects of Coenzyme Q*, Vol. 4, pp. 315–332, Elsevier Science Publishers B.V., 1984.

Ishihara, Y.; Uchida, Y.; Kitamura, S.; and Takaku, F. Effect of Coenzyme Q_{10}, a Quinone Derivative, on Guinea Pig Lung and Tracheal Tissue. *Arzneimittel-Forschung Drug Research* 35 (I), 6, 926–933, 1985.

Iwamoto, Yoshifumi; Nakamura, Ryo; and Folkers, Karl. Study of Periodontal Disease and Coenzyme Q. *Research Communications in Chemical Pathology and Pharmacology*, Vol. 11, No. 2, June 1975.

Iwamoto, Yoshifumi; Yamagami, Toru; and Folkers, Karl. Deficiency of Coenzyme Q_{10} in Hypertensive Rats and Reduction of Deficiency by Treatment with Coenzyme Q_{10}. *Biochemical and Biophysical Research Communications*, Vol. 58, No. 3, pp. 743–748, 1974.

Iwamoto, Yoshifumi; Watanabe, Tatsuo; et al. Clinical Effect of Coenzyme Q_{10} on Periodontal Disease. *Biomedical and Clinical Aspects* of Coenzyme Q, Vol. 3, pp. 109–119, Elsevier/ North-Holland Biomedical Press, 1981.

Judy, W.V.; Hall, J.H.; Toth, P.D.; and Folkers, K. Myocardial Effects of Co-Enzyme Q_{10} in Primary Heart Failure. *Biomedical and Clinical Aspects of Coenzyme Q*, Vol. 4, pp. 352–368, Elsevier Science Publishers B.V., 1984.

Judy, W.V.; Hall, J.H.; Dugan, W.; Toth, P.D.; and Folkers, K. Coenzyme Q_{10} Reduction of Adriamycin Cardiotoxicity. *Biomedical and Clinical Aspects of Coenzyme Q*, Vol. 4, pp. 231–241, Elsevier Science Publishers B.V., 1984.

Kamikawa, Tadishi; Kobayashi, Akira; Yamashita, Tetsuo; et al. Effects of Coenzyme Q_{10} on Exercise Tolerance in Chronic Stable Angina Pectoris. *American Journal of Cardiology* 56, pp. 247–251, 1985.

Kanazawa, Takemichi; Koh, Meikyu; Kato, Masashi; et al. A Study on Myocardial Energy Metabolism in Ischemic Heart Disease—The Effects of Large Dose Administration of CoQ_{10}. *Biomedical and Clinical Aspects of Coenzyme Q*, Vol. 4, pp. 273–280, Elsevier Science Publishers B.V., 1984.

Kantrowitz, Niki E., and Bristow, Michael R. Cardiotoxicity of Antitumor Agents. *Progress in Cardiovascular Diseases*, Vol. 27, No. 3, pp. 195–200, November/December 1984.

Katagiri, Takashi; Sasai, Yasufumi; Kobayashi, Youichi; et al. Protective Effect of Coenzyme Q_{10} on the Acute Ischemic Myocardial Injury. *Biomedical and Clinical Aspects of Coenzyme Q*, Vol. 3, pp. 349–359, Elsevier/North-Holland Biomedical Press, 1981.

Kawase, Ichiro; Niitani, Hisanobu; Saijo, Nagahiro; et al. Enhancing Effect of Coenzyme Q_{10} on Immunorestoration with Mycobacterium Bovis BCG in Tumor-Bearing Mice. *Gann* 69, pp. 493–497, August 1978.

Kayawake, Setsuo; Nakanishi, T.; Furukawa, K.; et al. The Protective Effect of Coenzyme Q_{10} upon the Jeopardized Myocardium. *Biomedical and Clinical Aspects of Coenzyme Q*, Vol. 4, pp. 173–179, Elsevier Science Publishers B.V., 1984.

Kent, Saul. *Your Personal Life-Extension Program*. William Morrow and Company, New York, 1985.

Kishi, Hiroe; Kanamori, Nobuhiro; Nishii, Satoshi; et al. Metabolism of Exogenous Coenzyme Q_{10} in Vivo and the Bioavailability of Coenzyme Q_{10} Preparations in Japan. *Biomedical and Clinical Aspects of Coenzyme Q*, Vol. 4, pp. 131–142, Elsevier Science Publishers B.V., 1984.

Kishi, Takeo; Makino, Kazuo; Okamato, Tadashi; et al. Inhibition of Myocardial Respiration by Psychotherapeutic Drugs and Prevention by Coenzyme Q. *Biomedical and Clinical Aspects of Coenzyme Q*, Vol. 2, pp. 139–154, Elsevier/North-Holland Biomedical Press, 1980.

Kishi, Takeo; Takahashi, Kyoko; Mayumi, Tadanori; and Hama Takao. Protective Effect of Coenzyme Q on Adriamycin Toxicity in Beating Heart Cells. *Biomedical and Clinical Aspects of Coenzyme Q*, Vol. 4, pp. 181–194, Elsevier Science Publishers B.V., 1984.

Kishi, Takeo; Watanabe, Tatsuo; and Folkers, Karl. Bioenergetics in Clinical Medicine XV. Inhibition of Coenzyme Q_{10}-Enzymes by Clinically Used Adrenergic Blockers of B(Beta)-Receptors. *Research Communications in Chemical Pathology and Pharmacology*, Vol. 17, No. 1, May 1977.

Kishimoto, Chiharu; Tamaki, Shunichi; Matsumori, Akira; et al. The Protection of Coenzyme Q_{10} Against Experimental Viral Myocarditis in Mice. *Japanese Circulation Journal*, Vol. 48, No. 12, pp. 1358–1361, December 1984.

Kitamura, Nobuo; Yamaguchi, Akimitsu; Otaki, Masami; et al. Myocardial Tissue Level of Coenzyme Q_{10} in Patients with Cardiac Failure. *Biomedical and Clinical Aspects of Coenzyme Q*, Vol. 4, pp. 243–252, Elsevier Science Publishers B.V., 1984.

Klein, Reinhild; Maisch, B.; Kochsiek, K.; and Berg, P.A. Demonstration of Organ Specific Antibodies against Heart Mitochondria (Anti-M7) in Sera From Patients with Some Forms of Heart Diseases. *Clinical Experimental Immunology* 58, pp. 283–392, 1984.

Kohli, Yoshihiro; Suto, Yoshimasa; and Kodama, Tadashi. Effect of Hypoxia on Acetic Acid Ulcer of the Stomach in Rats with or without Coenzyme Q_{10}. *Journal of Experimental Medicine*, Japan, Vol. 51, pp. 105–108, 1981.

Kondo et al. Method of Producing Coenzyme Q_{10} by Microorganisms. United States Patent # 3,769,170, Oct. 30, 1973.

Konishi, Takashi; Nakamura, Yasuyuki; Konishi, Tomotsugu; and Kawai, Chuichi. Improvement in Recovery of Left Ventricular Function During Reperfusion with Coenzyme Q_{10} in Isolated Working Rat Heart. *Cardiovascular Research*, Volume 19, No. 1, pp. 38–43, January 1985.

Kuratsu, Yoshiyuki; Hagino, Hiroshi; and Inuzuka, Keiichi. Effect of Ammonium Ion on Coenzyme Q_{10} Fermentation by Agrobacterium Species. *Agric. Biol. Chem.* 48 (5), pp. 1347–1348, 1984.

Langsjoen, P.H.; Vadhanavikit S.; and Folkers, K. Effective Treatment with Coenzyme Q_{10} of Patients with Chronic Myocardial Disease. *Drugs under Experimental and Clinical Research*, Vol. 11, No. 8, pp. 577–580, 1985.

Langsjoen, P.H.; Vadhanavikit, Surasi; and Folkers, Karl. Effective Treatment with Coenzyme Q_{10} of Patients with Myocardial Disease, Classes III and IV. 1984. Unpublished.

————. Response of Patients in Classes III and IV of Cardiomyopathy to Therapy in a Blind and Crossover Trial with Coenzyme Q_{10}. *Proceedings National Academy of Sciences*, Vol. 82, pp. 4240–4244, June 1985.

Lenaz, G. *Coenzyme Q: Biochemistry, Bioenergetics and Clinical Applications of Ubiquinone*. John Wiley & Sons, New York, 1985.

Lenaz, G.; Fato, R.; Degli Esposti, M.; et al. The Essentiality of Coenzyme Q for Bioenergetics and Clinical Medicine. *Drugs under Experimental and Clinical Research*, Vol. 11, No. 8, pp. 547–556, 1985.

Lenaz, G., and Parenti Castelli, G. Multiple Roles of Ubiquinone in Mammalian Cells. *Drugs Exptl. Res.* X(7), pp. 481–490, 1984.

Littarru, Gian Paolo; De Sole, Pasquale; Lippa, Silvio; and Oradei, Alessandro. Study of Quenching of Singlet Oxygen by Coenzyme Q_{10} in a System of Human Leucocytes.

Littarru, G.P., and Lippa, S. Coenzyme Q and Antioxidant Activity: Facts and Perspectives. *Drugs Exptl. Clin. Res.* X(7), pp. 491–496, 1984.

Littarru, G.P.; Lippa, S.; De Sole, P.; and Oradei, A. In Vitro Effect of Different Ubiquinones on the Scavenging of Biologically Generated O2. *Drugs under Experimental and Clinical Research*, Vol. 11, No. 8, pp. 529–532, 1985.

Loe, Harold. The Role of Bacteria in Periodontal Disease. *Bulletin of the World Health Organization* 59 (6), pp. 821–825, 1981.

Marubayashi, Seiji; Dohi, Kiyohiko; Yamada, Kazuo; and Kawasaki, Takashi. Changes in the Levels of Endogenous Coenzyme Q Homologs, Tocopherol, and Glutathione in Rat Liver after Hepatic Ischemia and Reperfusion, and the Effect of Pretreatment with Coenzyme Q_{10}. *Biochemica et Biophysica Acta* 797, pp. 1–9, Elsevier Science Publishers B.V., 1984.

Marubayashi, S.; Dohi, K.; Ezaki, H.; Yamada, K.; and Kawasaki, T. Preservation of Ischemic Liver Cell—Prevention of Damage by Coenzyme Q_{10}. *Transplantation Proceedings*, Vol. 15, No. 1, March 1983.

McCarty, Mark F. Towards a "Bio-Energy Supplement"—A Prototype for Functional Orthomolecular Supplementation. *Medical Hypotheses* 7, pp. 515–538, 1981.

———. Optimized Mitochondrial Function as a Nutritional Strategy in Cancer Immunotherapy. *Medical Hypotheses* 7, pp. 55–60, 1981.

Monden, M.; Toyoshima, K.; Gotoh, M.; et al. Effect of Coenzyme Q_{10} on Cadaveric Liver Transplantation in Dogs. *Transplantation Proceedings*, Vol. 16, No. 1, February 1984.

Mortensen, S.A.; Vadhanavikit, S.; Baandrup, U.; and Folkers, K. Long-Term Coenzyme Q_{10} Therapy: A Major Advance in the Management of Resistant Myocardial Failure. *Drugs under Experimental and Clinical Research*, Vol. 11, No.8, p. 581, 1985.

Mortensen, Svend Aage; Vadhanavikit, Surasi; and Folkers, Karl. Apparent Effectiveness of Coenzyme Q_{10} (CoQ) to Treat Patients with Cardiomyopathy and CoQ Levels in Blood and Endomycardial Biopsies. *Biomedical and Clinical Aspects of Coenzyme Q*, Vol. 4, pp. 391–402, Elsevier Science Publishers B.V., 1984.

Murakami, M.; Oketani, K.; Fujisaki, H.; et al. Antiulcer Effect of Geranylgeranylacetone, A New Acyclic Polyisoprenoid on Experimentally Induced Gastric and Duodenal Ulcers in Rats. *Arzneimittel-Forschung Drug Research* 31, (I), 5, pp. 799–804, 1981.

Murakami, Manabu; Oketani, Kiyoshi; Fujisaki, Hideaki; et al. Effect of Synthetic Acyclic Polyisoprenoids on the Cold-Restraint Stress Induced Gastric Ulcer in Rats. *Japan Journal of Pharmacology* 33, pp. 549–556, 1983.

Nagano, Makoto; Takahashi, Kaoru; Komori, Akihiko; et al. Effect of Coenzyme Q_{10} on Myocardial Function and Metabolism in Rat Heart-Lung Preparations. *Biomedical and Clinical Aspects of Coenzyme Q*, Vol. 4, pp. 121–129, Elsevier Science Publishers B.V., 1984.

Nakao, et al. Method for the Production of Coenzyme Q. United States Patent # 3,658,648, April 25, 1972.

Nohara, Ryuji; Yokode, Masayuki; Tanaka, Masaru; et al. Effect of CoQ_{10} on Cardiac Function. *Biomedical and Clinical Aspects of Coenzyme Q*, Vol. 4, pp. 343–352, Elsevier Science Publishers B.V., 1984.

Nakamura, Yoshiro; Takahashi, Masando; Hayashi, Junichi; et al. Protection of Ischemic Myocardium with Coenzyme Q_{10}. *Cardiovascular Research*, Vol. 16, No. 3, pp. 132–137, March 1982.

Nayler, Winifred G. The Use of Coenzyme Q_{10} to Protect Ischaemic Heart Disease. *Biomedical and Clinical Aspects of Coenzyme Q*, Vol. 2, pp. 409–424, Elsevier/North-Holland Biomedical Press, 1980.

Nobuyoshi, Masakiyo; Saito, Taro; Takahira, Hideo; et al. Levels of Coenzyme Q_{10} in Biopsies of Left Ventricular Muscle and Influence of Administration of Coenzyme Q_{10}. *Biomedical and Clinical Aspects of Coenzyme Q*, Vol. 4, pp. 221–229, Elsevier Science Publishers B.V., 1984.

Nohara, Ryuji; Yokode, Masayuki; Tanaka, Masaru; et al. Effect of CoQ_{10} on Cardiac Function. *Biomedical and Clinical Aspects of Coenzyme Q*, Vol. 4, pp. 343–352, Elsevier Science Publishers B.V., 1984.

Nohl, Hans, and Werner Jordan. The Biochemical Role of Ubiquinone and Ubiquinone-Derivatives in the Generation of Hydroxyl-Radicals from Hydrogen-Peroxide. *Oxygen Radicals in Chemistry and Biology*, Walter de Gruyter & Co., 1984.

Oda, T. Effect of Coenzyme Q_{10} on Stress-Induced Cardiac Dysfunction in Paediatric Patients with Mitral Valve Prolapse: A Study by Stress Echocardiography. *Drugs under Experimental and Clinical Research*, Vol. 11, No. 8, pp. 557–576, 1985.

Oda, Teiichi, and Hamamoto, Kunihiro. Effect of Coenzyme Q_{10} on the Stress-Induced Decrease of Cardiac Performance in Pediatric Patients with Mitral Valve Prolapse. *Japanese Circulation Journal*, Vol. 48, No. 12, p. 137, December 1984.

Okada, Ryozo; Kasuya, Hideaki; Ih, Seimei; and Ogawa, Masahiro. Histopathological Study of Adriamycin (ADR)-Cardiotoxicity in Rats and the Protective Effects of Beta-Blockade, Ca-Antagonist and CoQ_{10}. *Japanese Circulation Journal*, Vol. 47, No. 7, p. 830, 1983.

Okamoto, Kouji, and Ogura Ryohei. Effects of Vitamins on Lipid Peroxidation and Suppression of DNA Synthesis Induced by Adriamycin in Ehrlich Cells. *J. Nutr. Sci. Vitaminol.* 31, pp. 129–137, 1985.

Okamoto, T.; Fukui, K.; Nakamoto, M.; and Kishi T. High-Performance Liquid Chromatography of Coenzyme Q-Related Compounds and its

Application to Biological Materials. *Journal of Chromatography* 342, pp. 35–46, 1985.

Olson, Robert E., and Rudney, Harry. Biosynthesis of Ubiquinone. *Vitamins and Hormones*, Vol. 40, pp. 2–43, 1983.

Peterman, Thomas A.; Drotman, Peter D.; and Curran, James W. Epidemiology of the Acquired Immunodeficiency Syndrome (AIDS). *Epidemiologic Reviews*, Vol. 7, 1985.

Pouplard, A., and Emile, J. New Immunological Findings in Senile Dementia. *Interdisciplinary Topics in Gerentology*, Vol. 19, pp. 62–71, Karger, Basel 1985.

Regelson, William, and Sinex, Msarrott F. Intervention in the Aging Process, Part A: Quantitation, Epidemiology, and Clinical Research. *Enzyme Cofactors in Aging*, Karl Folkers, pp. 199–214, 1983.

Richardson, Philip C.; Baker, Lee E.; Folkers, Karl; et al. Clinical Studies on Coenzyme Q_{10} for Treatment of Cardiovascular Disease. *Biomedical and Clinical Aspects of Coenzyme Q*, Vol. 2, pp. 301–308, Elsevier/North-Holland Biomedical Press, 1980.

Roitt, Ivan M. *Essential Immunology*. Blackwell Scientific Publications, Oxford, England, 1971.

Rosen, Philip. Aging of the Immune System. *Medical Hypotheses* 18, pp. 157–161, 1985.

Saiki, I.; Tokushima, Y.; Nishimura, K.; and Azuma, I. Macrophage Activation with Ubiquinones and Their Related Compounds in Mice. *International Journal for Vitamin and Nutrition Research*, No. 3, pp. 312–320, 1983.

Sanma, Hideyuki, and Nakamura, Tetsuya. Effects of Adriamycin and Coenzyme Q_{10} on Leukotriene C-Like Substance Formation in the Guinea Pig Heart. *Biochemistry International*, Vol. 5, No. 5, pp. 617–627, November 1982.

Schmid, Rolf D. Biotechnology in Japan 1984. Part 1. Industrial Activities. *Appl. Michrobiol. Biotechnol* 22, pp. 157–164, 1985.

Schneeberger, W.; Zilliken F.; Moritz J.; et al. Clinical Studies with Coenzyme Q_{10} in Patients with Congestive Heart Failure. *Drugs Exptl. Clin. Res.* X(7), pp. 503–512, 1984.

Sevanian, Alex, and Hochstein, Paul. Mechanisms and Consequences of Lipid Peroxidation in Biological Systems. *Ann. Rev. Nutr.* 5, pp. 365–390, 1985.

Shizukuishi, Satosha; Inoshita, Eiji; Tsunemitsu, Akira; et al. Effect of Coenzyme Q_{10} on Experimental Periodontitis in Dogs. *Biomedical Research* 4 (1), pp. 33–40, 1983.

Simic, Michael G., and Hunter, Edward P.L. Interactions of Free Radicals and Antioxidants. *Radioprotectors and Anticarcinogens*, pp. 449–459, Academic Press, Inc., New York, 1983.

Sohal, R.S. Metabolic Rate, Free Radicals, and Aging. Free Radicals in Molecular Biology. *Aging and Disease*. Raven Press, New York, 1984.

Solani, G.; Ronca, G.; Bertelli, A. Inhibitory Effects of Several Anthracyclines on Mitochondrial Respiration and Coenzyme Q_{10} Protection. *Drugs under Experimental and Clinical Research*, Vol. 11, No. 8, pp. 533–538, 1985.

Sugimoto, Mineharu; Ideta, Toru; Imanishi, Koji; et al. Effect of Coenzyme Q_{10} (Ubiquinone) in Patients with Progressive Muscular Dystrophy and Other Neuromuscular Diseases. *Biomedical and Clinical Aspects of Coenzyme Q*, pp. 243–249, Elsevier/North-Holland Biomedical Press, 1977.

Sunamori, Makoto; Okamura, Takao; Amano, Jun; and Suzuki, Akio. Clinical Applications of Coenzyme Q to Coronary Artery Bypass Graft Surgery. *Biomedical and Clinical Aspects of Coenzyme Q*, Vol. 4, pp. 333–342, Elsevier Science Publishers B.V., 1984.

Suzuki, Noboru; Nakamura, Tetsuya; Ishida, Hideyuki; and Hosono, Kiyoshi. Protective Effect of Coenzyme Q_{10} against Hypoxic Cellular Damage. *Chem. Pharm. Bull.*, Vol. 33, pp. 2896–2903, 1985.

Takada, Masahiro; Yuzuriha, Teruaki; and Yamato, Chiyuki. Redox Levels of Intravenously Administered Coenzyme Q_{10} and Coenzyme Q_{10}-reducing Activity in Subcellular Fractions of Guinea Pig Liver. *J. Nutr. Sci. Vitaminol.*, Vol. 31, pp. 147–155, 1985.

Takada, Masahiro; Yuzuriha, Teruaki; Katayama, Kouichi; et al. Targeting of Coenzyme Q_{10} Solubilized with Soy Lecithin to Heart of Guinea Pigs. *J. Nutr. Sci. Vitaminol.*, Vol. 31, pp. 115–120, 1985.

Tanaka, Jiro; Tominaga, Ryuji; Yoshitoshi, Mochikazu; et al. Coenzyme Q_{10}: The Prophylactic Effect on Low Cardiac Output Following Cardiac Valve Replacement. *Annals of Thoracic Surgery*, Vol. 33, No. 2, February 1982.

Tengerdy, Robert P.; Mathias, Melvin M.; and Nockels, Cheryl F. Effect of Vitamin E on Immunity and Disease Resistance. *Vitamins, Nutrition and Cancer,* pp. 123–133, Karger, Basel, 1984.

Thaler-Dao, Helene; Crastes de Paulet, Andre; and Paoletti, Rodolfo. *Icosanoids and Cancer*. Raven Press, New York, 1982.

Thomson, R. H. *Naturally Occurring Quinones* (second edition). Academic Press, London, England, 1971.

Tsuyasaki, Teruo; Noro, Chuji; and Kikawada, Ryuichi. Mechanocardiography of Ischemic or Hypertensive Heart Failure. *Biomedical and Clinical Aspects of Coenzyme Q*, Vol. 2, pp. 273–288, Elsevier/North-Holland Biomedical Press, 1980.

Van Gaal, Luc; De Leeuw, Ivo; Vadhanavikit, Surasi; and Folkers, Karl. Exploratory Study of Coenzyme Q_{10} in Obesity. *Biomedical and Clinical Aspects of Coenzyme Q*, Vol. 4, pp. 369–373, Elsevier Science Publishers B.V., 1984.

Vanfraechem, J.H.P.; Picaluasa, C.; and Folkers, K. Coenzyme Q_{10} and Physical Performance in Myocardial Failure. *Biomedical and Clinical Aspects of Coenzyme Q*, Vol. 4, pp. 281–289, Elsevier Science Publishers B.V., 1984.

Vanfraechem, J.H.P., and Folkers, Karl. Coenzyme Q_{10} and Physical Performance. *Biomedical and Clinical Aspects of Coenzyme Q*, Vol. 3, pp. 235–241, Elsevier/North-Holland Biomedical Press, 1981.

Weksler, Marc E., and Siskind, Gregory W. The Cellular Basis of Immune Senescence. Monographs in Developmental Biology, Vol. 17, pp. 110–121, 1984.

Wilkinson, Edward G.; Arnold, Ralph M.; Karl Folkers; et al. Bioenergetics in Clinical Medicine. II. Adjunctive Treatment with Coenzyme Q in Periodontal Therapy. *Research Communications in Chemical and Clinical Pharmacology*, Vol. 12, No. 1, September 1975.

Wilkinson, E.G., and Folkers, Karl. Measuring Changes in the Health of the Human Periodontium and other Oral Tissues. *Biomedical and Clinical Aspects of Coenzyme Q*, Vol. 3., pp. 93–102, Elsevier/North-Holland Biomedical Press, 1981.

Wilkinson, E.G.; Arnold, R.M.; and Folkers, Karl. Treatment Of Periodontal and other Soft Tissue Disease of the Oral Cavity with Coenzyme Q. *Biomedical and Clinical Aspects of Coenzyme Q*, pp. 251–266, Elsevier/North-Holland Biomedical Press, 1977.

Wilkinson R.F., and Folkers, K. The Treatment of Benign Mucous Pemphigoid with Coenzyme Q_{10}. *Biomedical and Clinical Aspects of Coenzyme Q*, Vol. 3, pp. 103–108, Elsevier/ North-Holland Biomedical Press, 1981.

Yamada, Kazuo; Tatsukawa, Yorimitsu; Takenaka, Masaharu; et al. Coenzyme Q and the Restoration of Functions in the Ischemic Kidney and Brain. *Biomedical and Clinical Aspects of Coenzyme Q*, Vol. 2, pp. 123–132, Elsevier/North-Holland Biomedical Press, 1980.

Yamakawa, Katsutoshi; Fukuta, Shinji; Kimura, Yoshio; et al. Circulating Anti-Heart Antibodies in Heart Diseases Detected Using an Immunofluorescent Technique. *Japanese Circulation Journal*, Vol. 47, No. 10, pp. 1173–1178, October 1983.

Yamagami, Toru; Shibata, Nobuhiko; and Folkers, Karl. Bioenergetics in Clinical Medicine. Studies on Coenzyme Q_{10} and Essential Hypertension. *Research Communications in Chemical Pathology and Pharmacology*, Vol. 11, No. 2, pp. 273–288, June 1975.

Yamagami, Toru; Shibata, Nobuhiko; and Folkers, Karl. Bioenergetics in XClinical Medicine. VIII. Administration of Coenzyme Q_{10} to Patients with Essential Hypertension. *Research Communications in Chemical Pathology and Pharmacology*. Vol. 14, No. 4, pp. 721–727, August 1976.

Yamagami, Toru; Shibata, Nobuhiko; and Folkers, Karl. Study of Activities of the Succinate Dehydrogenase-Coenzyme Q Reductase in Leucocytes of Patients with Controlled Hypertension. *Journal Of Medicine*, Vol. 9, No. 2, pp. 145–155, 1978.

Yamagami, Toru; Takagi, Satoko; Akagami, Hirotaka; et al. Correlation between Serum Coenzyme Q Levels and Succinate Dehydrogenase Coenzyme Q Reductase Activity in Cardiovascular Diseases and the Influence of Coenzyme Q Administration. *Biomedical and Clinical Aspects of Coenzyme Q*, Vol. 4, pp. 253–262, Elsevier Science Publishers B.V., 1984.

Yamasawa, Ikuhiro; Nohara, Yoshitugu; Konno, Senichiro; et al. Experimental Studies on Effects of Coenzyme Q_{10} on Ischemic Myocardium. *Biomedical and Clinical Aspects of Coenzyme Q*, Vol. 2, pp. 333–345, Elsevier/North-Holland Biomedical Press, 1980.

Yazaki, Yoshio; Nagai, Ryozo; and Chiu, Chung-Cheng. Preservation of Ischemic Myocardium by Coenzyme Q_{10}; Assessment by Serial Changes in Serum Cardiac Myosin Light Chain II. *Biomedical and Clinical Aspects of Coenzyme Q*, Vol. 4, pp. 163–170, Elsevier Science Publishers B.V., 1984.

Yuzuriha, Teruaki; Takada, Masairo; and Katayama, Kouichi. Transport of Coenzyme Q_{10} from the Liver to other Tissues after Intravenous Administration to Guinea Pigs. *Biochimica et Biophysica Acta* 759, pp. 286–291, 1983.

Zbinden, Gerhard; Bachmann, Elisabeth; and Bolliger, Heidi. Study of Coenzyme Q in Toxicity of Adriamycin. *Clinical Aspects of Coenzyme Q*, pp. 219–228, Elsevier/North-Holland Biomedical Press, 1977.

Zilliken, Fritz; Moritz, Joachim; Muller-Steinwachs, Johannes; et al. Double Blind Clinical Study with CoQ_{10} in Patients with a Low Cardiac Function. *Biomedical and Clinical Aspects of Coenzyme Q*, Vol. 4, pp. 425–426, Elsevier Science Publishers B.V., 1984.

Index

ABOUT THE AUTHORS

DR. EMILE G. BLIZNAKOV, a leading American expert on the immune system and aging, has more than twenty-five years of research experience in biomedicine, including medical immunology, microbiology, gerontology, neurochemistry and the field of cancer. His studies have been conducted not only in the United States but in the Soviet Union and Bulgaria where he was born and educated. Dr. Bliznakov is credited with the publication of more than eighty papers in prestigious scientific journals and medical textbooks worldwide, and has formally presented his work in over twenty foreign countries in Europe, Asia, Australia and South America. Dr. Bliznakov was formerly President of the New England Institute and is presently President, Scientific Director and Member of the Board of Trustees of the Ridgefield, Connecticut-based Lupus Research Institute. A member of numerous American medical institutions and societies, Dr. Bliznakov also has the honor of being elected a Fellow of the world-renowned Royal Society of Tropical Medicine and Hygiene, London, England. He resides in Connecticut.

GERALD L. HUNT is a former international newspaper journalist turned author. He specializes in medical and health-related topics and is the author of four books. Born and educated in Yorkshire, England, Hunt was a reporter and feature writer for the prestigious *Daily Mail* of London, and later deputy bureau chief for that paper based in Belfast, Northern Ireland, during the height of the country's troubles in the late 60s and early 70s. Since moving to the United States in 1973, Hunt has worked as a staff reporter and writer for several major magazines and news journals. He is also a former correspondant for a number of leading British newspapers including *The Times, The Observer,* the *Daily Telegraph* and the *Daily Express.* He is presently founder and President of Northern News Service International and lives in Connecticut.

Printed in the United States
by Baker & Taylor Publisher Services